LOW SODIUM

FOOD LIST 2024

The comprehensive guide to what food to avoid and eat with ingredient list for High Blood Pressure, Stroke and Heart Failure

Jane Galaz

Table of Contents

Introduction..**3**

Understanding Sodium and Its Effects on Health.......................7

Importance of a Low Sodium Diet...11

How to Use This Guide...15

Chapter 1: Understanding Sodium...................................**18**

What is Sodium?... 18

Sodium's Role in the Body..22

Health Risks of Excess Sodium... 26

Recommended Sodium Intake Levels.................................... 30

Chapter 2: Benefits of a Low Sodium Diet......................**33**

Improved Heart Health.. 33

Lower Blood Pressure.. 37

Enhanced Kidney Function...41

Overall Wellness...45

Chapter 3: Reading Nutrition Labels.............................. **49**

Identifying Sodium Content... 49

Hidden Sources of Sodium...53

Tips for Choosing Low Sodium Products................................57

Chapter 4: Foods to Eat... **60**

Fruits and Vegetables...60

Whole Grains...70

Protein Sources.. 79

Dairy Alternatives...87

Snacks and Convenience Foods............................ 102

Chapter 5: Foods to Avoid.................................. **116**

Processed and Packaged Foods...........................116

Snacks and Junk Food..................................... 124

Condiments and Sauces.................................... 130

Baked Goods... 140

Chapter 6: Low Sodium Meal Planning.................. **148**

Weekly Meal Planning Tips................................. 148

Creating Balanced, Low Sodium Meals.................. 151

Grocery Shopping Strategies............................... 154

Chapter 7: Cooking Techniques............................**157**

Using Fresh Herbs and Spices............................. 157

Flavor Enhancers Without Sodium.........................161

Cooking Methods That Preserve Flavor.................. 164

Chapter 8: Sample Meal Plans............................. **168**

7Day Low Sodium Meal Plan................................168

Recipes for Breakfast..171

Lunch Recipes..179

Dinner Recipes... 187

Snack Ideas...195

Chapter 9: Dining Out Tips...................................**210**

Choosing Low Sodium Options at Restaurants...................... 210

Customizing Orders to Reduce Sodium....................213

Understanding Restaurant Menus........................... 216

Chapter 10: Maintaining a Low Sodium Lifestyle....................219

Strategies for LongTerm Success............................ 219

Staying Motivated and Consistent........................... 223

Monitoring Your Progress....................................... 227

CONCLUSION...231

Introduction

In the bustling city of Ever well, there lived a spirited woman named Clara. Clara had always been the life of the party, known for her vibrant personality and infectious laughter. But recently, her boundless energy had started to wane.

She often felt fatigued, and her blood pressure was alarmingly high. A visit to the doctor confirmed her worst fears: Clara needed to make drastic changes to her diet to manage her health, particularly her sodium intake.

Determined to reclaim her vitality, Clara embarked on a quest for knowledge. She scoured the internet for resources, but the overwhelming amount of conflicting information left her feeling more confused than ever.

Just when she was about to lose hope, Clara stumbled upon the "Low Sodium Food List 2024." Intrigued by its promise to simplify her dietary journey, she decided to give it a try.

As Clara delved into the pages of the guide, she found herself pleasantly surprised.

The "Low Sodium Food List 2024" was not just a list of foods to eat and avoid; it was a comprehensive roadmap to a healthier lifestyle.

The first chapter provided a clear understanding of sodium's role in the body and the health risks associated with excessive intake. Clara appreciated the straightforward explanations and felt more informed about why she needed to reduce her sodium consumption.

The guide's second chapter outlined the numerous benefits of a low sodium diet, from improved heart health to better kidney function. Clara felt a renewed sense of purpose as she read about how these changes could enhance her overall well-being.

She was particularly inspired by the success stories of others who had transformed their lives through low sodium eating.

One of the most valuable sections for Clara was the chapter on reading nutrition labels. She had always found food labels confusing, but the guide broke down the process into simple steps, teaching her how to identify hidden sources of sodium.

Armed with this knowledge, Clara felt more confident navigating the grocery store aisles.

The "Low Sodium Food List 2024" also offered a plethora of delicious and creative recipes. Clara discovered new favorites, like herbed quinoa salad and roasted vegetable medley.

The guide included tips on using fresh herbs and spices to enhance flavor without relying on salt. Clara enjoyed experimenting in the kitchen, and her meals became not only healthier but also more flavorful and exciting.

Meal planning had always been a challenge for Clara, but the guide provided practical advice on creating balanced, low sodium meals. Clara learned how to prepare her meals in advance, saving time and ensuring she always had healthy options on hand.

The sample meal plans and grocery shopping strategies were particularly helpful, making the transition to a low sodium lifestyle seamless.

Dining out had been another source of stress for Clara, but the guide offered valuable tips on choosing low sodium options at restaurants. Clara learned how to customize her orders and ask for dressings and sauces on the side. These small changes made a big difference, allowing her to enjoy social outings without compromising her health goals.

As Clara continued to follow the "Low Sodium Food List 2024," she noticed remarkable improvements in her health. Her blood pressure stabilized, her energy levels soared, and she felt more vibrant than she had in years. Clara was no longer just surviving; she was thriving.

Reflecting on her journey, Clara realized that purchasing the "Low Sodium Food List 2024" had been one of the best decisions she had ever made. The guide had provided her with the knowledge, tools, and inspiration she needed to take control of her health.

Clara's story is a testament to the power of informed dietary choices and the transformative impact of the "Low Sodium Food List 2024." For anyone looking to improve their health and embrace a low sodium lifestyle, this guide is an invaluable companion on the path to wellness.

Understanding Sodium and Its Effects on Health

Sodium is an essential mineral that plays a vital role in various bodily functions. It helps regulate fluid balance, nerve function, and muscle contractions. Despite its importance, consuming too much sodium can lead to significant health issues.

In modern diets, high sodium intake is often due to the prevalence of processed and packaged foods, which are typically loaded with sodium for preservation and flavor enhancement. Understanding the impact of sodium on health is crucial, especially for those who need to adhere to a low sodium diet.

Excessive sodium intake is closely linked to high blood pressure, a major risk factor for heart disease and stroke. When there is too much sodium in the bloodstream, it can cause the body to retain water, increasing the volume of blood.

This higher blood volume puts extra pressure on blood vessels, leading to hypertension. Managing sodium intake is essential for maintaining healthy blood pressure levels and reducing the risk of cardiovascular complications.

Kidney function is also affected by sodium levels. The kidneys play a crucial role in filtering excess sodium from the body. However, when sodium intake is consistently high, the kidneys may struggle to keep up, leading to fluid retention and swelling.

Over time, this can impair kidney function and increase the risk of chronic kidney disease. Adopting a low sodium diet can help alleviate the burden on the kidneys and support their optimal function.

Moreover, high sodium intake is associated with an increased risk of osteoporosis. Sodium can cause calcium to be excreted in the urine, leading to a gradual loss of calcium from bones.

This can weaken bones over time and increase the likelihood of fractures and osteoporosis, particularly in older adults. A low sodium diet can help preserve bone health by minimizing calcium loss and promoting better bone density.

Stomach health is another area where sodium has a significant impact. High sodium diets are linked to an increased risk of gastric cancer.

The exact mechanism is not fully understood, but it is believed that high sodium levels can damage the stomach lining and increase susceptibility to infection by Helicobacter pylori, a bacteria associated with gastric ulcers and cancer.

Reducing sodium intake can help protect the stomach lining and lower the risk of these serious conditions.

Additionally, reducing sodium intake can have immediate benefits, such as reduced bloating and water retention. Many people experience bloating and discomfort from consuming too much sodium, as the body retains extra water to balance the sodium levels.

By lowering sodium intake, individuals can often see a noticeable reduction in bloating, leading to increased comfort and a better overall feeling of well-being.

The Low Sodium Food List 2024 serves as a valuable tool for individuals aiming to manage their sodium intake effectively. It provides a comprehensive guide to foods that are low in sodium, helping individuals make informed choices about their diet.

By understanding the effects of sodium on health and utilizing resources like the Low Sodium Food List 2024, people can take proactive steps to improve their health, prevent disease, and enhance their quality of life.

Adopting a low sodium lifestyle is not just about cutting out salt; it's about embracing a healthier, more balanced way of eating that supports overall wellness.

Importance of a Low Sodium Diet

The significance of a low sodium diet cannot be overstated, particularly for those aiming to enhance their overall health and well-being. Sodium, an essential mineral, plays a crucial role in various bodily functions, including fluid balance, nerve transmission, and muscle function.

However, excessive sodium intake can lead to severe health issues, making it imperative to monitor and reduce sodium consumption. The Low Sodium Food List 2024 provides an invaluable resource for individuals striving to manage their sodium intake effectively, offering a comprehensive guide to make healthier dietary choices.

One of the primary benefits of adhering to a low sodium diet is the positive impact it has on cardiovascular health. High sodium intake is closely linked to hypertension, or high blood pressure, which is a major risk factor for heart disease and stroke.

By reducing sodium consumption, individuals can lower their blood pressure, thereby decreasing the likelihood of cardiovascular complications.

The Low Sodium Food List 2024 offers an extensive selection of heart-healthy foods that are low in sodium, enabling individuals to make informed decisions that support their cardiovascular health.

Beyond heart health, a low sodium diet is also beneficial for kidney function. The kidneys play a vital role in regulating sodium levels in the body, and excessive sodium intake can put undue stress on these organs.

Over time, this can lead to kidney damage and decreased kidney function. By following the recommendations in the Low Sodium Food List 2024, individuals can help protect their kidneys and maintain optimal kidney health. The guide includes a variety of kidney-friendly foods that are low in sodium, making it easier to adhere to a diet that supports renal function.

Another critical aspect of a low sodium diet is its role in preventing water retention and bloating. High sodium levels can cause the body to retain excess water, leading to uncomfortable bloating and swelling, particularly in the extremities.

Reducing sodium intake can help alleviate these symptoms and promote a more comfortable, balanced state of hydration.

The Low Sodium Food List 2024 highlights foods that are naturally low in sodium and less likely to cause water retention, allowing individuals to feel lighter and more at ease.

Adopting a low sodium diet can also enhance overall well-being by promoting better dietary habits. Processed and packaged foods, which are often high in sodium, tend to be less nutritious than whole, unprocessed foods. By focusing on low sodium options, individuals are more likely to consume a diet rich in fruits, vegetables, whole grains, and lean proteins.

These nutrient-dense foods provide essential vitamins and minerals that support overall health and vitality. The Low Sodium Food List 2024 serves as a valuable tool for identifying these nutritious options and incorporating them into daily meals.

Moreover, a low sodium diet can contribute to weight management. Many high sodium foods are also high in calories and unhealthy fats, contributing to weight gain and obesity. By choosing low sodium alternatives, individuals can reduce their calorie intake and make healthier food choices that support weight loss or maintenance.

The Low Sodium Food List 2024 includes a wide range of low-calorie, low-sodium foods that can aid in achieving and maintaining a healthy weight, further promoting overall health.

Ultimately, the importance of a low sodium diet extends beyond the prevention of specific health conditions. It represents a commitment to a healthier lifestyle and the proactive management of one's well-being.

The Low Sodium Food List 2024 provides a comprehensive and practical guide for anyone looking to reduce their sodium intake and improve their health.

By offering a wealth of information on low sodium foods and practical tips for incorporating them into everyday meals, this guide empowers individuals to take control of their diet and make positive changes that will benefit their health for years to come.

How to Use This Guide

To make the most of the Low Sodium Food List 2024, begin by familiarizing yourself with the foundational information provided in the early chapters. These sections cover the importance of a low sodium diet, the health risks associated with high sodium intake, and the benefits of reducing sodium consumption.

By understanding the underlying principles, you can appreciate the necessity of incorporating low sodium foods into your daily routine and how this lifestyle change can significantly enhance your overall well-being.

As you dive into the guide, take time to learn how to read nutrition labels effectively. This skill is crucial for identifying hidden sources of sodium in processed and packaged foods. The guide breaks down the process into simple steps, making it easy for you to decipher labels and make informed choices.

Practice this newfound knowledge during your grocery shopping trips to ensure you select products that align with your low sodium goals.

The food lists are designed to help you easily distinguish between foods to eat and foods to avoid. Spend time reviewing these lists to familiarize yourself with the options available. By incorporating a variety of low sodium foods into your meals, you can create a balanced and enjoyable diet.

Experiment with different ingredients and recipes provided in the guide to keep your meals interesting and satisfying. This will help you stay committed to your low sodium lifestyle.

Meal planning is an integral part of maintaining a low sodium diet. Use the sample meal plans and grocery shopping tips in the guide to streamline your weekly preparation. Planning your meals in advance not only saves time but also reduces the likelihood of resorting to high sodium convenience foods.

Batch cooking and storing meals in portioned containers can make it easier to stick to your dietary plan, even on busy days.

Dining out while adhering to a low sodium diet can be challenging, but the guide offers valuable strategies to navigate restaurant menus. Learn how to identify low sodium options and customize your orders to fit your dietary needs.

The tips provided will empower you to make healthier choices without sacrificing flavor or enjoyment. With these strategies, you can confidently enjoy social meals while staying true to your low sodium goals.

Staying hydrated is essential for managing sodium levels, and the guide emphasizes the importance of choosing appropriate beverages. It provides recommendations for low sodium drinks and explains how to avoid those that may contain hidden sodium. By following these guidelines, you can support your overall health and enhance the effectiveness of your low sodium diet.

Regularly consulting the guide and staying updated with new information will help you maintain a successful low sodium lifestyle. Use the resources and tools provided, such as apps and online communities, to stay motivated and connected with others on a similar journey.

Continuous learning and adaptation are key to long-term success. Embrace the Low Sodium Food List 2024 as your trusted companion, guiding you towards a healthier, more balanced life.

Chapter 1: Understanding Sodium

What is Sodium?

Sodium is a mineral and an essential electrolyte that plays a crucial role in maintaining several physiological functions in the body. It is primarily found in the blood and the fluid surrounding cells, where it helps regulate fluid balance, blood pressure, and the function of nerves and muscles.

Sodium facilitates the transmission of nerve impulses and is vital for muscle contractions, including those of the heart. Despite its essential functions, the body only requires a small amount of sodium to perform these tasks effectively.

In our daily diet, sodium is most commonly consumed in the form of sodium chloride, also known as table salt. Salt is a widespread ingredient used in cooking and food preservation, contributing to the flavor and shelf life of many foods.

However, sodium is also present in various forms in processed and packaged foods, making it easy to consume more than the recommended amount. High sodium intake is linked to numerous health issues, particularly cardiovascular diseases, due to its impact on blood pressure.

Excessive sodium intake leads to an imbalance in the body's fluid regulation. When there is too much sodium in the bloodstream, the body retains water to dilute it, increasing the volume of blood. This heightened blood volume exerts additional pressure on the walls of blood vessels, leading to high blood pressure, also known as hypertension.

Over time, this increased pressure can damage the blood vessels, heart, and kidneys, contributing to the risk of heart disease, stroke, and kidney failure.

Managing sodium intake is crucial for individuals with certain health conditions, such as hypertension, heart disease, and chronic kidney disease. For these individuals, reducing sodium consumption can help manage symptoms and prevent complications.

It can also benefit the general population by promoting heart health and preventing the development of related diseases.

Awareness and education about sodium's role and its effects are essential steps toward adopting a healthier lifestyle.

The human body requires only a minimal amount of sodium to function correctly, typically less than 500 milligrams per day. However, the average sodium consumption in many countries far exceeds this amount, often due to the prevalence of processed and restaurant foods.

Foods high in sodium include canned soups, deli meats, fast foods, and snack items such as chips and pretzels. Even foods that may not taste salty, such as bread and cereals, can contain significant amounts of sodium.

Adopting a low sodium diet involves more than just reducing table salt usage. It requires careful consideration of all food sources, reading nutrition labels, and making informed choices about the foods we eat.

Fresh fruits and vegetables, lean proteins, and whole grains are typically lower in sodium and can be enjoyed more freely. Additionally, cooking at home allows for better control over sodium content, using herbs and spices to enhance flavor without the need for added salt.

Understanding sodium and its impact on health is the first step toward making better dietary choices. By recognizing the sources of sodium in our diet and the importance of moderation, we can take proactive measures to protect our health.

The Low Sodium Food List 2024 serves as a valuable resource in this journey, offering guidance on selecting low sodium foods and providing practical tips for maintaining a balanced, heart-healthy diet.

Sodium's Role in the Body

Sodium plays a crucial role in the body's overall function and well-being. It is an essential electrolyte that helps regulate fluid balance, ensuring that cells receive the right amount of hydration. This balance is vital for maintaining blood pressure and supporting the proper functioning of muscles and nerves.

Sodium allows the body to conduct electrical signals, which are necessary for muscle contractions, including those of the heart. By maintaining these signals, sodium helps keep the heart rhythm steady and muscles responsive.

The body's fluid balance is intricately tied to sodium levels. When sodium levels are in the correct range, the body can efficiently manage the amount of water inside and outside cells. This regulation is crucial for preventing dehydration and maintaining healthy blood volume and pressure.

When you consume sodium, it is absorbed into the bloodstream and helps retain water, which in turn maintains blood pressure. However, an imbalance, particularly excess sodium, can disrupt this delicate system, leading to health issues like hypertension.

Sodium also plays a role in nutrient absorption in the digestive tract. It assists in the absorption of nutrients such as glucose and amino acids. These nutrients are essential for energy production and cell repair. Sodium facilitates the transport of these molecules across cell membranes, ensuring that the body can effectively utilize the food consumed.

Without adequate sodium, the body would struggle to absorb these critical nutrients efficiently, impacting overall health and energy levels.

Despite its importance, it is easy for sodium levels to become too high due to dietary choices. Processed foods, fast foods, and many packaged items contain high amounts of sodium, which can lead to an overconsumption.

When sodium intake exceeds the recommended levels, the kidneys, which regulate sodium in the body, may not be able to excrete the excess efficiently. This can lead to water retention, increased blood volume, and subsequently, higher blood pressure.

Persistent high blood pressure is a major risk factor for heart disease, stroke, and kidney damage.

Maintaining the appropriate balance of sodium is thus critical for health. For individuals with conditions such as hypertension, kidney disease, or heart failure, managing sodium intake is particularly important.

These conditions can be exacerbated by high sodium levels, leading to further health complications. A low sodium diet can help mitigate these risks by reducing the strain on the cardiovascular system and kidneys, promoting better overall health outcomes.

Understanding sodium's role in the body underscores the importance of monitoring and controlling sodium intake. The Low Sodium Food List 2024 serves as a valuable resource in this regard, helping individuals identify foods that are safe to eat and those to avoid.

By adhering to a low sodium diet, you can support your body's natural functions, maintain healthy blood pressure, and reduce the risk of serious health issues. The guide empowers you to make informed dietary choices that align with your health goals.

Incorporating a variety of low sodium foods into your diet not only supports your health but also enhances your culinary experience.

Fresh fruits and vegetables, lean proteins, and whole grains are excellent choices that provide essential nutrients without the excess sodium.

By following the recommendations in the Low Sodium Food List 2024, you can enjoy flavorful, nutritious meals while maintaining optimal sodium levels.

This approach ensures that you can live a healthier, more balanced life, free from the complications associated with high sodium intake.

Health Risks of Excess Sodium

Excessive sodium intake poses significant health risks that can affect various aspects of your well-being. One of the most immediate and well-known dangers is the impact on blood pressure. Consuming too much sodium causes the body to retain water, which increases the volume of blood in your bloodstream.

This added volume exerts extra pressure on the walls of your arteries, leading to elevated blood pressure. Hypertension, or high blood pressure, is a major risk factor for heart disease and stroke, two of the leading causes of death worldwide.

Beyond its impact on blood pressure, excess sodium can strain the cardiovascular system. The heart must work harder to pump the increased volume of blood, which can lead to an enlarged heart and weakened heart muscle over time.

This condition, known as left ventricular hypertrophy, can reduce the heart's efficiency and increase the risk of heart failure. Furthermore, high sodium levels can contribute to the buildup of plaque in the arteries, a condition called atherosclerosis.

This narrowing and hardening of the arteries restrict blood flow and can result in heart attacks and strokes.

Kidney function is also adversely affected by high sodium intake. The kidneys play a crucial role in filtering excess sodium out of the bloodstream and excreting it through urine.

However, consistently high levels of sodium can overwhelm the kidneys, impairing their ability to function properly. This can lead to chronic kidney disease, a progressive condition that can eventually result in kidney failure.

People with existing kidney issues are particularly vulnerable, as their kidneys are already compromised and less capable of handling excess sodium.

High sodium intake is associated with an increased risk of osteoporosis. Sodium can cause the body to excrete more calcium in the urine. This calcium loss can weaken bones over time, making them more susceptible to fractures.

Maintaining strong bones requires a careful balance of minerals, and excessive sodium disrupts this balance, potentially leading to decreased bone density and osteoporosis, especially in older adults.

Another concerning aspect of high sodium consumption is its effect on fluid balance and swelling. Excess sodium can cause fluid retention, leading to swelling in the hands, feet, and ankles. This condition, known as edema, can be uncomfortable and sometimes painful.

In severe cases, fluid retention can accumulate in the lungs, causing pulmonary edema, which impairs breathing and requires immediate medical attention.

Excessive sodium intake can also have indirect effects on overall health by influencing dietary habits. High sodium foods are often processed and low in essential nutrients, leading to poor dietary quality.

This can result in deficiencies in vital nutrients such as potassium, calcium, and magnesium, which are important for maintaining heart and bone health.

A diet high in processed, sodium-laden foods often means lower consumption of fruits, vegetables, and whole grains, further exacerbating health risks.

Finally, it's important to recognize the cumulative effect of high sodium intake over time. While occasional indulgence in salty foods might not cause immediate harm, consistent overconsumption can lead to chronic health issues.

Reducing sodium intake by following guidelines like those in the Low Sodium Food List 2024 can significantly lower these health risks. Adopting a low sodium diet helps in managing blood pressure, protecting cardiovascular and kidney health, maintaining bone density, and promoting overall well-being.

By understanding and mitigating the health risks associated with excess sodium, individuals can take proactive steps toward a healthier future.

Recommended Sodium Intake Levels

Sodium intake levels are crucial for maintaining optimal health, and understanding the recommended guidelines can help you make better dietary choices. The average adult should aim to consume no more than 2,300 milligrams of sodium per day, which is approximately equivalent to one teaspoon of salt.

However, for individuals with specific health conditions such as hypertension, heart disease, or chronic kidney disease, the recommended intake is even lower, typically around 1,500 milligrams per day.

Adhering to these guidelines can be challenging, especially given the high sodium content in many processed and packaged foods. It's essential to become mindful of sodium intake and learn how to manage it effectively.

Most people consume far more sodium than necessary, often without realizing it. This excessive intake can lead to serious health issues, including high blood pressure, stroke, and heart disease.

One of the key strategies for managing sodium intake is to focus on fresh, whole foods rather than processed options.

Fresh fruits and vegetables, lean meats, and whole grains naturally contain lower levels of sodium compared to their processed counterparts. By incorporating these foods into your diet, you can significantly reduce your sodium consumption and improve your overall health.

Reading nutrition labels is another important aspect of managing sodium intake. Nutrition labels provide detailed information about the sodium content of packaged foods, helping you make informed choices.

Look for products labeled as "low sodium," "reduced sodium," or "no salt added." These labels indicate that the products contain less sodium than their regular counterparts, making them better choices for a low sodium diet.

When preparing meals at home, use herbs, spices, and other flavor enhancers to reduce your reliance on salt. Fresh herbs like basil, cilantro, and parsley, as well as spices like cumin, turmeric, and paprika, can add depth and flavor to your dishes without increasing sodium levels.

Additionally, using lemon juice, vinegar, and garlic can enhance the taste of your food naturally.

Dining out can pose challenges for those trying to limit their sodium intake, but it is possible with careful planning. Many restaurants offer nutritional information on their menus or websites, allowing you to choose lower sodium options.

Requesting that your food be prepared without added salt, asking for sauces and dressings on the side, and avoiding high sodium condiments can help you stay within your recommended sodium intake levels.

Monitoring and adjusting your sodium intake is an ongoing process that requires awareness and commitment. Regularly checking your blood pressure and discussing your diet with a healthcare provider can help you stay on track.

By following the recommended sodium intake levels and making conscious dietary choices, you can manage your sodium intake effectively, reduce the risk of related health issues, and promote overall well-being.

The Low Sodium Food List 2024 serves as a valuable resource in this journey, providing guidance and support to help you achieve and maintain a healthy, balanced diet.

Chapter 2: Benefits of a Low Sodium Diet

Improved Heart Health

Embracing a low sodium diet can significantly improve heart health by reducing the strain on the cardiovascular system. High sodium intake is closely linked to elevated blood pressure, a major risk factor for heart disease and stroke.

By reducing your sodium consumption, you can lower your blood pressure, decreasing the risk of these serious health conditions. The Low Sodium Food List 2024 serves as an essential guide to help you make informed dietary choices that support heart health.

The reduction of sodium in your diet helps to balance fluid levels in the body. Excess sodium causes the body to retain water, increasing blood volume and putting extra pressure on the blood vessels.

This added strain can lead to hypertension and damage to the cardiovascular system over time. By opting for low sodium foods, you can maintain proper fluid balance, easing the burden on your heart and blood vessels.

Adopting a low sodium diet also promotes better function of the endothelium, the inner lining of the blood vessels. High sodium levels can impair endothelial function, leading to reduced elasticity of the arteries and increased arterial stiffness.

This condition can exacerbate high blood pressure and contribute to the development of atherosclerosis, a condition where plaque builds up in the arteries. A low sodium diet helps preserve endothelial health, enhancing arterial flexibility and overall cardiovascular function.

Weight management is another critical aspect of heart health that can be positively influenced by a low sodium diet. Many high sodium foods are also high in calories and unhealthy fats, contributing to weight gain and obesity, which are risk factors for heart disease.

By focusing on low sodium, nutrient-dense foods such as fruits, vegetables, whole grains, and lean proteins, you can better manage your weight. This not only reduces the strain on your heart but also lowers the risk of other related conditions like diabetes and metabolic syndrome.

Additionally, a low sodium diet can reduce the risk of developing left ventricular hypertrophy, a condition where the heart's left ventricle thickens and enlarges due to high blood pressure. This condition can lead to heart failure if left unchecked.

By maintaining a diet low in sodium, you can help prevent the onset of left ventricular hypertrophy and promote a healthier heart structure.

Implementing a low sodium diet encourages healthier eating habits overall. When you reduce sodium, you often increase your intake of fresh, whole foods that are naturally low in sodium, such as fruits, vegetables, and whole grains.

These foods are rich in essential nutrients, antioxidants, and fiber, all of which contribute to cardiovascular health.

The Low Sodium Food List 2024 provides a comprehensive selection of these heart-healthy foods, making it easier to adopt and maintain a beneficial dietary pattern.

The long-term commitment to a low sodium diet fosters a sustainable approach to heart health.

As you become more accustomed to preparing and enjoying low sodium meals, your taste preferences will adjust, making it easier to stick with the diet.

Over time, these dietary changes can lead to significant improvements in heart health, enhancing your quality of life and longevity.

By following the guidance of the Low Sodium Food List 2024, you are taking proactive steps towards a healthier heart and a healthier you.

Lower Blood Pressure

A key benefit of following a low sodium diet is the significant reduction in blood pressure, which can greatly improve overall cardiovascular health. High blood pressure, or hypertension, is a major risk factor for heart disease and stroke, and it often results from excessive sodium intake.

By lowering sodium consumption, you can effectively manage and reduce your blood pressure levels, thereby decreasing the strain on your heart and blood vessels.

When you consume less sodium, your body retains less water. This reduction in fluid retention helps lower the volume of blood that your heart has to pump, leading to a decrease in blood pressure.

The Low Sodium Food List 2024 provides a comprehensive guide to foods that are naturally low in sodium, helping you make better dietary choices that support this important health goal. Incorporating these foods into your daily meals can create a positive impact on your blood pressure levels.

Adopting a low sodium diet not only helps in reducing blood pressure but also enhances the effectiveness of blood pressure medications.

For individuals who are on antihypertensive drugs, a low sodium diet can amplify the benefits of these medications, often allowing for lower doses and fewer side effects.

This synergistic effect makes it easier to manage blood pressure consistently and effectively, contributing to better long-term health outcomes.

In addition to the direct impact on blood pressure, a low sodium diet often encourages the consumption of more potassium-rich foods, such as fruits and vegetables.

Potassium helps balance the effects of sodium and supports overall cardiovascular health by aiding in the relaxation of blood vessel walls and promoting the excretion of sodium through urine.

The Low Sodium Food List 2024 highlights numerous potassium-rich, low sodium options that can enhance your diet and further support blood pressure management.

The psychological benefits of lowering blood pressure should not be overlooked. Managing hypertension can reduce anxiety and stress associated with health concerns. Knowing that you are taking proactive steps to improve your health can provide peace of mind and enhance your overall quality of life.

The Low Sodium Food List 2024 offers practical advice and easy-to-follow recipes that make it simpler to maintain a low sodium diet, helping you stay committed to your health goals without feeling overwhelmed.

As you continue to follow a low sodium diet, you may notice additional health benefits such as reduced risk of kidney disease, improved bone health, and a lower likelihood of developing stomach cancer.

These improvements are all interconnected with the reduction of blood pressure and overall sodium intake. By sticking to the guidelines provided in the Low Sodium Food List 2024, you are not only working towards lowering your blood pressure but also supporting your general health and well-being.

Maintaining a low sodium diet is a sustainable and effective approach to managing blood pressure and enhancing overall health. The Low

Sodium Food List 2024 serves as an invaluable resource, offering clear guidance and practical tools to help you make informed dietary choices.

By embracing this lifestyle change, you can enjoy the multitude of benefits that come with lower blood pressure, leading to a healthier and more vibrant life.

Enhanced Kidney Function

Enhanced kidney function is one of the most significant benefits of adhering to a low sodium diet, and this improvement plays a crucial role in overall health. The kidneys are responsible for filtering waste products, excess fluids, and electrolytes, such as sodium, from the bloodstream.

By reducing your sodium intake, you can alleviate the stress on these vital organs, allowing them to function more efficiently and effectively. This is particularly important for individuals with existing kidney conditions, as it helps prevent further damage and supports the maintenance of optimal kidney health.

High sodium levels in the diet can lead to an increase in blood pressure, which in turn places additional strain on the kidneys. When blood pressure rises, the blood vessels in the kidneys can become damaged, reducing their ability to filter blood properly.

A low sodium diet helps to regulate blood pressure, thereby protecting the kidneys from this type of damage. This protective effect is crucial for preventing the progression of chronic kidney disease and reducing the risk of kidney failure.

Another key aspect of improved kidney function on a low sodium diet is the reduction in fluid retention. High sodium intake can cause the body to retain excess water, leading to swelling and increased workload for the kidneys.

By cutting back on sodium, you can help your body maintain a proper fluid balance, easing the burden on your kidneys. This not only enhances kidney function but also contributes to overall comfort and well-being by reducing symptoms such as bloating and edema.

A low sodium diet can also positively impact the production and excretion of urine. With a lower sodium intake, the kidneys can better regulate the balance of electrolytes in the body, which is essential for maintaining healthy urine production.

This improved balance helps to prevent complications such as kidney stones, which can form when there are imbalances in substances like calcium, oxalate, and uric acid in the urine.

By maintaining a low sodium diet, you support the kidneys in keeping these substances at healthy levels.

In addition to protecting against kidney stones, a low sodium diet supports the kidneys' ability to manage and excrete waste products efficiently. When sodium levels are high, the kidneys have to work harder to eliminate excess sodium and other waste products.

This increased workload can lead to a decline in kidney function over time. By reducing sodium intake, you lessen the strain on your kidneys, enabling them to perform their waste removal duties more effectively and sustain their function for a longer period.

Maintaining a low sodium diet also helps to reduce the risk of proteinuria, a condition where excess protein is found in the urine. Proteinuria is often an early sign of kidney damage, as it indicates that the kidneys' filtering mechanisms are not working properly.

By keeping sodium intake low, you can help protect these filtering mechanisms and reduce the likelihood of proteinuria, thereby preserving kidney health.

Overall, enhanced kidney function is a pivotal benefit of a low sodium diet, contributing to improved health outcomes and quality of life.

By following the guidelines and recommendations in the Low Sodium Food List 2024, you can support your kidneys in their vital role of maintaining fluid and electrolyte balance, filtering waste, and regulating blood pressure.

This proactive approach to diet and health empowers you to take control of your well-being and enjoy the long-term benefits of optimal kidney function.

Overall Wellness

Adopting a low sodium diet offers numerous benefits that contribute to overall wellness, making it a vital component of a healthy lifestyle. One of the most significant advantages is the positive impact on heart health.

Excessive sodium intake is closely linked to high blood pressure, a major risk factor for heart disease and stroke. By reducing sodium consumption, you can lower your blood pressure, which in turn decreases the strain on your heart and arteries.

This simple dietary change can lead to a significant reduction in the risk of cardiovascular events, promoting long-term heart health.

Beyond heart health, a low sodium diet also supports better kidney function. The kidneys play a crucial role in regulating sodium balance in the body, and high sodium intake can overburden these vital organs.

When you consume less sodium, your kidneys don't have to work as hard to eliminate excess sodium, reducing the risk of kidney damage and chronic kidney disease.

This is especially important for individuals who already have compromised kidney function, as managing sodium intake can help slow the progression of kidney-related issues.

Another benefit of a low sodium diet is the potential for improved bone health. High sodium intake can lead to increased calcium loss through urine, which can weaken bones over time and increase the risk of osteoporosis.

By reducing sodium consumption, you help preserve bone density and support overall skeletal health. This is particularly beneficial for older adults and those at risk of osteoporosis, as maintaining strong bones is essential for preventing fractures and maintaining mobility.

A low sodium diet can also enhance your overall energy levels and reduce the feeling of bloating. Excess sodium can cause your body to retain water, leading to a feeling of puffiness and sluggishness.

By cutting back on sodium, you can help your body release excess fluid, which can make you feel lighter and more energetic. This improvement in energy levels can have a positive impact on your daily activities, making it easier to stay active and engaged in your favorite pursuits.

Mental clarity and cognitive function can also benefit from a low sodium diet. High blood pressure, often caused by excessive sodium intake, is associated with cognitive decline and an increased risk of dementia.

By managing your sodium intake and maintaining healthy blood pressure levels, you can support better brain health and potentially reduce the risk of cognitive issues as you age. This connection between diet and mental wellness underscores the importance of a holistic approach to health.

Weight management is another area where a low sodium diet can be beneficial. Many high-sodium foods are also high in calories and unhealthy fats, contributing to weight gain and obesity. By focusing on low sodium foods, you are more likely to choose fresh, whole foods that are nutrient-dense and lower in calories.

This shift can support weight loss and help you maintain a healthy weight, further reducing the risk of associated health problems such as diabetes and metabolic syndrome.

In summary, the benefits of a low sodium diet extend far beyond the reduction of sodium itself.

By embracing the principles outlined in the Low Sodium Food List 2024, you can enjoy improved heart health, better kidney function, enhanced bone strength, increased energy levels, better cognitive function, and effective weight management.

These comprehensive benefits contribute to your overall wellness, making a low sodium diet a cornerstone of a healthier, more balanced lifestyle.

Chapter 3: Reading Nutrition Labels

Identifying Sodium Content

When aiming to maintain a low sodium diet, one of the most crucial skills to develop is the ability to accurately identify sodium content in foods. This process begins with understanding how to read nutrition labels effectively.

The Nutrition Facts label, found on packaged foods, provides essential information about the nutrient content, including sodium. By paying close attention to this label, you can make informed choices that support your dietary goals.

The sodium content on a nutrition label is typically listed in milligrams (mg) per serving. It's important to note the serving size and the number of servings per container, as these can significantly impact your sodium intake.

A seemingly low sodium food can become a high sodium food if consumed in larger quantities than the serving size indicated.

Always compare the serving size on the label to the amount you actually eat to get an accurate picture of your sodium consumption.

When reading the sodium content, be aware of the daily recommended limit, which for most adults is 2,300 milligrams, with an ideal target of 1,500 milligrams for those with specific health concerns like hypertension.

Understanding these benchmarks helps you gauge whether a food item fits into your daily sodium allowance. Foods labeled as "low sodium" contain 140 milligrams of sodium or less per serving, making them suitable choices for a low sodium diet.

Hidden sources of sodium can also be a challenge. Ingredients such as monosodium glutamate (MSG), baking soda, baking powder, and sodium nitrate are common culprits.

These additives contribute to the overall sodium content but are not always immediately obvious. Additionally, terms like "sodium," "soda," and "Na" (the chemical symbol for sodium) can indicate the presence of sodium.

Familiarizing yourself with these terms can help you spot hidden sources of sodium in ingredient lists.

Processed and packaged foods often contain high levels of sodium for preservation and flavor enhancement. Foods such as canned soups, frozen meals, processed meats, and snack foods are notorious for their high sodium content.

When possible, opt for fresh, whole foods that are naturally low in sodium. If you do purchase processed foods, look for products specifically labeled as "low sodium," "very low sodium," or "no salt added." These options can help you manage your sodium intake more effectively.

Learning to identify sodium content is not just about avoiding high sodium foods but also about making smarter choices overall. For instance, when choosing between different brands of the same product, compare their sodium levels and opt for the one with lower sodium content.

Over time, these small adjustments can make a significant difference in your overall sodium intake and contribute to better health outcomes.

By mastering the skill of reading nutrition labels and identifying sodium content, you empower yourself to take control of your diet.

This proactive approach is essential for maintaining a low sodium lifestyle and achieving your health goals.

With the knowledge and strategies provided in the Low Sodium Food List 2024, you can navigate the grocery store with confidence, make healthier choices, and enjoy the benefits of a reduced sodium diet.

Hidden Sources of Sodium

When managing a low sodium diet, it's crucial to be aware of hidden sources of sodium that can easily sneak into your meals. Sodium is often present in foods that might not taste particularly salty, which can make it challenging to keep your intake within recommended limits.

Understanding these hidden sources is essential for maintaining a healthy diet and achieving your low sodium goals.

Processed and packaged foods are among the most common hidden sources of sodium. Items like canned soups, sauces, and ready-to-eat meals often contain high levels of sodium to enhance flavor and preserve shelf life.

Even seemingly healthy options like canned vegetables and legumes can be significant contributors to your daily sodium intake. Always check the nutrition labels of these products, paying close attention to the sodium content per serving.

Breads and bakery products are another surprising source of sodium. Although they might not taste salty, many types of bread, rolls, and bakery items contain added sodium as a leavening agent or preservative. This includes not only white and whole wheat bread but also bagels, muffins, and even some pastries.

When selecting these items, look for those labeled as low sodium or check the ingredient list to find options with reduced salt content.

Deli meats and processed meats are also notorious for their high sodium levels. Items like ham, bacon, sausages, and deli slices are often cured, smoked, or seasoned with salt.

These meats can quickly add a significant amount of sodium to your diet, even in small portions. Opt for fresh, unprocessed meats whenever possible, and if you do choose deli meats, look for those specifically labeled as low sodium.

Condiments and sauces are often overlooked as major sources of sodium. Common condiments like ketchup, mustard, soy sauce, and salad dressings can contain high amounts of sodium. Additionally, marinades, gravies, and seasoning blends are frequently loaded with salt.

To manage your sodium intake, consider using these items sparingly or seek out low sodium versions. Homemade alternatives using fresh herbs and spices can also be a flavorful substitute.

Cheese and dairy products, while important sources of calcium and protein, can also contribute to your sodium intake. Many types of cheese, particularly processed and hard cheeses, are high in sodium.

Be mindful of the types and amounts of cheese you consume, and opt for low sodium varieties when available. Additionally, check the labels on other dairy products like cottage cheese and yogurt, as these can also vary widely in sodium content.

Restaurant and takeout foods are often significant sources of hidden sodium. Even meals that appear healthy, such as salads or grilled items, can be laden with sodium from dressings, sauces, and seasoning blends used in preparation.

When dining out, ask for nutrition information if available and request that your food be prepared without added salt. Being proactive about your choices can help you manage your sodium intake more effectively.

Finally, be cautious with snacks and convenience foods. Items like chips, pretzels, crackers, and even some sweets can contain unexpected amounts of sodium.

These foods are often consumed in larger quantities, making it easy to exceed your daily sodium limit. Choosing low sodium snack options or making your own snacks at home can help you stay on track with your dietary goals.

By being vigilant about hidden sources of sodium and making informed choices, you can successfully manage your sodium intake and support your overall health.

Tips for Choosing Low Sodium Products

When selecting low sodium products, understanding how to read and interpret nutrition labels is crucial. The first step is to familiarize yourself with the serving size listed on the label.

Many products contain multiple servings, and the sodium content is often listed per serving. Ensure you calculate the total sodium intake based on the amount you actually consume to avoid underestimating your sodium intake.

Next, focus on the Percent Daily Value (%DV) for sodium. This percentage indicates how much of the recommended daily sodium intake is provided by one serving of the product.

As a general rule, aim for products that contain 5% or less of the daily value per serving, which is considered low. Items with 20% or more per serving are considered high in sodium and should be limited or avoided if possible.

Ingredients lists are another critical component of nutrition labels. Sodium can be present in various forms, including sodium chloride, sodium bicarbonate, and monosodium glutamate (MSG). Familiarize yourself with these terms and scan the ingredients list for them.

Additionally, be aware of words like "brined," "cured," "smoked," and "pickled," which often indicate higher sodium content due to the preservation process.

Processed and packaged foods are notorious for their hidden sodium content. When choosing such products, look for labels that specify "low sodium," "reduced sodium," or "no salt added." Be cautious, however, as "reduced sodium" only means that the product contains at least 25% less sodium than the regular version.

It does not necessarily mean the product is low in sodium overall. Always check the actual sodium content on the nutrition label to make an informed decision.

One effective strategy for reducing sodium intake is to opt for fresh, whole foods whenever possible. Fresh fruits, vegetables, lean meats, and whole grains generally contain less sodium compared to processed counterparts.

When buying canned or frozen vegetables, choose those labeled "no salt added" or rinse them thoroughly before cooking to remove some of the sodium.

Similarly, when purchasing meats, opt for fresh, unprocessed cuts rather than those that have been salted, smoked, or cured.

Another tip is to be mindful of condiments and sauces, which can be significant sources of hidden sodium. Items such as soy sauce, ketchup, salad dressings, and pre-made marinades often contain high levels of sodium.

Option for low sodium or homemade versions of these products, and use herbs, spices, and vinegar to add flavor to your meals instead. Reading labels on condiments is just as important as reading them on other food products.

Lastly, take advantage of the wealth of resources available to help you make better choices. Many grocery stores now provide low sodium product lists, and there are numerous apps designed to help you track and manage your sodium intake.

By consistently applying these tips and staying informed, you can effectively reduce your sodium consumption and improve your overall health. Embrace the Low Sodium Food List 2024 as a valuable tool in your journey towards a healthier, low sodium lifestyle.

Chapter 4: Foods to Eat

Fruits and Vegetables

In the context of a low sodium diet, fruits and vegetables play a vital role. They are naturally low in sodium and packed with essential nutrients.

Here is a comprehensive table listing 15 fruits and vegetables, along with their ingredients, instructions for preparation, nutritional information, serving size, and cooking time.

Food Item	Ingredients	Instructions	Nutritional Information (per serving)	Serving Size	Cooking Time
Apples	1 medium apple	Wash, core, and slice. Serve fresh or with a dip of	Calories: 95, Sodium: 2mg, Fiber: 4g, Sugar: 19g	1 medium apple	None

Food Item	Ingredients	Instructions	Nutritional Information (per serving)	Serving Size	Cooking Time
		your choice.			
Blueberries	1 cup fresh blueberries	Rinse under cold water. Serve fresh or add to yogurt or cereal.	Calories: 84, Sodium: 1mg, Fiber: 4g, Sugar: 15g	1 cup	None
Strawberries	1 cup fresh strawberries	Rinse under cold water, hull, and slice. Enjoy fresh or	Calories: 49, Sodium: 1mg, Fiber: 3g, Sugar: 7g	1 cup	None

Food Item	Ingredients	Instructions	Nutritional Information (per serving)	Serving Size	Cooking Time
		in a salad.			
Oranges	1 medium orange	Peel and segment. Serve fresh or in a fruit salad.	Calories: 62, Sodium: 0mg, Fiber: 3g, Sugar: 12g	1 medium orange	None
Grapes	1 cup seedless grapes	Rinse under cold water. Serve fresh or freeze for a cool treat.	Calories: 62, Sodium: 2mg, Fiber: 1g, Sugar: 16g	1 cup	None

Food Item	Ingredients	Instructions	Nutritional Information (per serving)	Serving Size	Cooking Time
Carrots	1 cup baby carrots	Rinse under cold water. Serve fresh or steam for 5-7 minutes until tender.	Calories: 50, Sodium: 42mg, Fiber: 3.5g, Sugar: 6g	1 cup	5-7 minutes
Bell Peppers	1 medium bell pepper	Wash, core, and slice. Serve fresh in salads or sauté for	Calories: 24, Sodium: 2mg, Fiber: 2g, Sugar: 3g	1 medium bell pepper	5-7 minutes

Food Item	Ingredients	Instructions	Nutritional Information (per serving)	Serving Size	Cooking Time
		5-7 minutes.			
Broccoli	1 cup broccoli florets	Steam for 5-7 minutes or roast in the oven at 400°F for 20 minutes.	Calories: 55, Sodium: 40mg, Fiber: 5g, Sugar: 2g	1 cup	5-7 minutes
Spinach	1 cup fresh spinach	Rinse under cold water. Serve fresh in salads or sauté for	Calories: 7, Sodium: 24mg, Fiber: 1g, Sugar: 0g	1 cup	3-5 minutes

Food Item	Ingredients	Instructions	Nutritional Information (per serving)	Serving Size	Cooking Time
		3-5 minutes.			
Cucumbers	1 medium cucumber	Wash and slice. Serve fresh in salads or as a snack with dip.	Calories: 16, Sodium: 2mg, Fiber: 1g, Sugar: 2g	1 medium cucumber	None
Tomatoes	1 medium tomato	Wash and slice. Serve fresh in salads, sandwiches, or salsa.	Calories: 22, Sodium: 6mg, Fiber: 1.5g, Sugar: 3g	1 medium tomato	None

Food Item	Ingredients	Instructions	Nutritional Information (per serving)	Serving Size	Cooking Time
Zucchini	1 medium zucchini	Wash and slice. Sauté for 5-7 minutes or grill for 10 minutes.	Calories: 33, Sodium: 2mg, Fiber: 2g, Sugar: 4g	1 medium zucchini	5-7 minutes
Pineapple	1 cup fresh pineapple chunks	Peel, core, and cut into chunks. Serve fresh or in fruit salads.	Calories: 82, Sodium: 2mg, Fiber: 2g, Sugar: 16g	1 cup	None

Food Item	Ingredients	Instructions	Nutritional Information (per serving)	Serving Size	Cooking Time
Mango	1 medium mango	Peel, slice, and serve fresh or in smoothies.	Calories: 99, Sodium: 2mg, Fiber: 2.6g, Sugar: 23g	1 medium mango	None
Kale	1 cup chopped kale	Rinse under cold water. Serve fresh in salads or sauté for 5-7 minutes.	Calories: 33, Sodium: 25mg, Fiber: 2g, Sugar: 0g	1 cup	5-7 minutes

Incorporating these fruits and vegetables into your diet can help you manage your sodium intake while enjoying a variety of flavors and textures.

Each item listed is naturally low in sodium and can be prepared quickly and easily, making them convenient choices for a healthy, low sodium lifestyle.

Whole grains are a vital component of a low sodium diet, providing essential nutrients, fiber, and sustained energy.

Below is a detailed guide to 15 whole grains, including ingredients, instructions, nutritional information, serving size, and cooking time.

Whole Grain	Ingredients	Instructions	Nutritional Information (per serving)	Serving Size	Cooking Time
Brown Rice	1 cup brown rice, 2 cups water	Rinse rice. Boil water, add rice, reduce heat, cover, simmer for 45 minutes.	Calories: 215, Protein: 5g, Carbs: 45g, Fiber: 4g, Sodium: 10mg	1 cup	45 minutes

Whole Grain	Ingredients	Instructions	Nutritional Information (per serving)	Serving Size	Cooking Time
Quinoa	1 cup quinoa, 2 cups water	Rinse quinoa. Boil water, add quinoa, cover, reduce heat, simmer for 15 mins.	Calories: 222, Protein: 8g, Carbs: 39g, Fiber: 5g, Sodium: 9mg	1 cup	15 minutes
Barley	1 cup barley, 3 cups water	Boil water, add barley, reduce heat, cover,	Calories: 193, Protein: 3.5g, Carbs: 44g, Fiber: 6g,	1 cup	45-50 minutes

Whole Grain	Ingredients	Instructions	Nutritional Information (per serving)	Serving Size	Cooking Time
		simmer for 45-50 minutes.	Sodium: 5mg		
Bulgur	1 cup bulgur, 2 cups water	Boil water, add bulgur, cover, simmer for 10-12 minutes.	Calories: 151, Protein: 5.6g, Carbs: 34g, Fiber: 8g, Sodium: 10mg	1 cup	10-12 minutes
Farro	1 cup farro, 3 cups water	Boil water, add farro, reduce heat, simmer	Calories: 170, Protein: 6g, Carbs: 35g, Fiber: 5g,	1 cup	30-40 minutes

Whole Grain	Ingredients	Instructions	Nutritional Information (per serving)	Serving Size	Cooking Time
		for 30-40 minutes.	Sodium: 5mg		
Millet	1 cup millet, 2.5 cups water	Boil water, add millet, cover, simmer for 20-25 minutes.	Calories: 207, Protein: 6g, Carbs: 41g, Fiber: 2g, Sodium: 3mg	1 cup	20-25 minutes
Oats (rolled)	1 cup oats, 2 cups water	Boil water, add oats, reduce heat, simmer for 5-7 minutes.	Calories: 154, Protein: 6g, Carbs: 27g, Fiber: 4g, Sodium: 1mg	1 cup	5-7 minutes

Whole Grain	Ingredients	Instructions	Nutritional Information (per serving)	Serving Size	Cooking Time
Teff	1 cup teff, 3 cups water	Boil water, add teff, reduce heat, simmer for 20 minutes.	Calories: 255, Protein: 10g, Carbs: 50g, Fiber: 7g, Sodium: 20mg	1 cup	20 minutes
Amaranth	1 cup amaranth, 3 cups water	Boil water, add amaranth, reduce heat, simmer for 20-25 minutes.	Calories: 251, Protein: 9g, Carbs: 46g, Fiber: 5g, Sodium: 15mg	1 cup	20-25 minutes

Whole Grain	Ingredients	Instructions	Nutritional Information (per serving)	Serving Size	Cooking Time
Spelt	1 cup spelt, 2.5 cups water	Boil water, add spelt, reduce heat, simmer for 25-30 minutes.	Calories: 246, Protein: 10g, Carbs: 51g, Fiber: 8g, Sodium: 7mg	1 cup	25-30 minutes
Sorghum	1 cup sorghum, 3 cups water	Boil water, add sorghum, reduce heat, simmer for 50-60 minutes.	Calories: 180, Protein: 5g, Carbs: 39g, Fiber: 6g, Sodium: 5mg	1 cup	50-60 minutes

Whole Grain	Ingredients	Instructions	Nutritional Information (per serving)	Serving Size	Cooking Time
Rye Berries	1 cup rye berries, 4 cups water	Boil water, add rye berries, reduce heat, simmer for 50-60 minutes.	Calories: 335, Protein: 10g, Carbs: 72g, Fiber: 25g, Sodium: 4mg	1 cup	50-60 minutes
Kamut	1 cup kamut, 3 cups water	Soak overnight, boil water, add kamut, simmer for 40-60 minutes.	Calories: 251, Protein: 11g, Carbs: 53g, Fiber: 7g, Sodium: 4mg	1 cup	40-60 minutes

Whole Grain	Ingredients	Instructions	Nutritional Information (per serving)	Serving Size	Cooking Time
Freekeh	1 cup freekeh, 2.5 cups water	Boil water, add freekeh, reduce heat, simmer for 20 minutes.	Calories: 200, Protein: 7g, Carbs: 41g, Fiber: 8g, Sodium: 10mg	1 cup	20 minutes
Buckwheat Groats	1 cup buckwheat, 2 cups water	Boil water, add buckwheat, cover, simmer for 15-20 minutes.	Calories: 155, Protein: 5g, Carbs: 33g, Fiber: 5g, Sodium: 1mg	1 cup	15-20 minutes

Whole grains offer numerous health benefits, including high fiber content, essential vitamins, and minerals while being naturally low in sodium.

By incorporating these grains into your diet, you can enjoy a variety of delicious, nutritious meals that support your low sodium lifestyle. Each grain provides unique flavors and textures, making your meals diverse and exciting.

Protein Sources

Incorporating protein sources that are low in sodium is essential for maintaining a healthy diet.

Here is a detailed table of 15 protein sources, including ingredients, instructions, nutritional information, serving size, and cooking time.

Protein Source	Ingredients	Instructions	Nutritional Information	Serving Size	Cooking Time
1. Chicken Breast	1 boneless, skinless chicken breast	Grill or bake until fully cooked, about 20-25 minutes at 375°F.	Calories: 165, Protein: 31g, Sodium: 60mg	4 oz	25 minutes
2. Turkey Breast	1 boneless, skinless turkey breast	Roast at 350°F for 25-30 minutes, or until	Calories: 135, Protein: 25g,	4 oz	30 minutes

Protein Source	Ingredients	Instructions	Nutritional Information	Serving Size	Cooking Time
		internal temperature reaches 165°F.	Sodium: 50mg		
3. Tofu	1 cup firm tofu	Press tofu to remove excess water, then grill or stir-fry for 5-7 minutes.	Calories: 176, Protein: 20g, Sodium: 15mg	1 cup	7 minutes
4. Tempeh	1 cup tempeh	Slice and steam for 10 minutes, then sauté or	Calories: 320, Protein: 31g, Sodium: 9mg	1 cup	17 minutes

Protein Source	Ingredients	Instructions	Nutritional Information	Serving Size	Cooking Time
		grill for an additional 5-7 minutes.			
5. Lentils	1 cup dried lentils	Rinse and cook in boiling water for 20-25 minutes, until tender.	Calories: 230, Protein: 18g, Sodium: 4mg	1 cup cooked	25 minutes
6. Quinoa	1 cup quinoa	Rinse quinoa and cook in 2 cups of water for 15-20 minutes,	Calories: 222, Protein: 8g, Sodium: 13mg	1 cup cooked	20 minutes

Protein Source	Ingredients	Instructions	Nutritional Information	Serving Size	Cooking Time
		until water is absorbed.			
7. Black Beans	1 cup dried black beans	Soak overnight, then cook in boiling water for 60-90 minutes, until tender.	Calories: 227, Protein: 15g, Sodium: 1mg	1 cup cooked	90 minutes
8. Chickpeas	1 cup dried chickpeas	Soak overnight, then cook in boiling water for 60-90	Calories: 269, Protein: 14.5g, Sodium: 6mg	1 cup cooked	90 minutes

Protein Source	Ingredients	Instructions	Nutritional Information	Serving Size	Cooking Time
		minutes, until tender.			
9. Salmon	4 oz salmon fillet	Grill, bake, or broil for 10-12 minutes, until fully cooked.	Calories: 206, Protein: 22g, Sodium: 50mg	4 oz	12 minutes
10. Cod	4 oz cod fillet	Bake at 375°F for 15-20 minutes, until flaky and opaque.	Calories: 90, Protein: 20g, Sodium: 55mg	4 oz	20 minutes

Protein Source	Ingredients	Instructions	Nutritional Information	Serving Size	Cooking Time
11. Eggs	2 large eggs	Boil for 9-12 minutes, scramble, or poach as desired.	Calories: 140, Protein: 12g, Sodium: 140mg	2 large eggs	12 minutes
12. Cottage Cheese	1 cup low sodium cottage cheese	Eat as is, or add to salads and snacks.	Calories: 206, Protein: 27g, Sodium: 29mg	1 cup	N/A
13. Greek Yogurt	1 cup plain Greek yogurt	Enjoy plain or with fresh fruit and nuts.	Calories: 100, Protein: 10g, Sodium: 50mg	1 cup	N/A

Protein Source	Ingredients	Instructions	Nutritional Information	Serving Size	Cooking Time
14. Edamame	1 cup edamame	Boil in water for 5-7 minutes, until tender.	Calories: 188, Protein: 18g, Sodium: 9mg	1 cup cooked	7 minutes
15. Almonds	1/4 cup unsalted almonds	Eat raw or roasted as a snack.	Calories: 207, Protein: 8g, Sodium: 0mg	1/4 cup	N/A

These protein sources are excellent options for maintaining a low sodium diet while ensuring adequate protein intake. Each item listed provides essential nutrients and can be easily incorporated into a variety of meals to keep your diet both balanced and enjoyable.

By following these simple instructions and nutritional guidelines, you can support your overall health and adhere to your low sodium dietary needs.

Dairy Alternatives

When following a low sodium diet, finding suitable dairy alternatives can be essential for maintaining nutritional balance while adhering to dietary restrictions.

Here is a comprehensive table of 15 dairy alternatives, including ingredients, instructions, nutritional information, serving size, and cooking time.

Dairy Alternative	Ingredients	Instructions	Nutritional Information	Serving Size	Cooking Time
Almond Milk	1 cup raw almonds, 4 cups water, 1 tsp vanilla extract (optional)	Soak almonds overnight. Drain and blend with water until smooth. Strain through a nut milk bag. Add vanilla extract if desired.	Calories: 40, Protein: 1g, Carbs: 2g, Fiber: 1g, Sugars: 1g, Fat: 3g, Sodium: 30mg, Potassium: 50mg	1 cup	10 minutes

Dairy Alternative	Ingredients	Instructions	Nutritional Information	Serving Size	Cooking Time
Soy Milk	1 cup soybeans, 4 cups water, 1 tsp vanilla extract (optional)	Soak soybeans overnight. Drain and blend with water until smooth. Strain through a nut milk bag. Boil for 10 minutes, then cool. Add vanilla	Calories: 80, Protein: 7g, Carbs: 4g, Fiber: 1g, Sugars: 1g, Fat: 4g, Sodium: 45mg, Potassium: 100mg	1 cup	20 minutes

Dairy Alternative	Ingredients	Instructions	Nutritional Information	Serving Size	Cooking Time
		extract if desired.			
Oat Milk	1 cup rolled oats, 4 cups water, 1 tsp vanilla extract (optional)	Blend oats and water until smooth. Strain through a nut milk bag. Add vanilla extract if desired.	Calories: 120, Protein: 3g, Carbs: 24g, Fiber: 2g, Sugars: 5g, Fat: 2g, Sodium: 60mg, Potassium: 130mg	1 cup	10 minutes
Coconut Milk	1 cup shredded coconut,	Blend shredded coconut	Calories: 45, Protein:	1 cup	10 minutes

Dairy Alternative	Ingredients	Instructions	Nutritional Information	Serving Size	Cooking Time
	4 cups water	and water until smooth. Strain through a nut milk bag.	0g, Carbs: 2g, Fiber: 0g, Sugars: 0g, Fat: 5g, Sodium: 15mg, Potassium: 50mg		
Rice Milk	1 cup cooked white rice, 4 cups water	Blend cooked rice and water until smooth. Strain through a	Calories: 120, Protein: 1g, Carbs: 23g, Fiber: 0g, Sugars: 10g, Fat:	1 cup	10 minutes

Dairy Alternative	Ingredients	Instructions	Nutritional Information	Serving Size	Cooking Time
		nut milk bag.	2g, Sodium: 60mg, Potassium: 30mg		
Cashew Milk	1 cup raw cashews, 4 cups water	Soak cashews for 2 hours. Drain and blend with water until smooth. Strain if desired.	Calories: 50, Protein: 1g, Carbs: 2g, Fiber: 0g, Sugars: 1g, Fat: 4g, Sodium: 20mg, Potassium: 50mg	1 cup	5 minutes

Dairy Alternative	Ingredients	Instructions	Nutritional Information	Serving Size	Cooking Time
Hemp Milk	1/2 cup hemp seeds, 4 cups water, 1 tsp vanilla extract (optional)	Blend hemp seeds and water until smooth. Strain through a nut milk bag. Add vanilla extract if desired.	Calories: 60, Protein: 3g, Carbs: 1g, Fiber: 1g, Sugars: 0g, Fat: 5g, Sodium: 10mg, Potassium: 110mg	1 cup	5 minutes
Macadamia Milk	1 cup raw macadamia nuts, 4 cups	Soak macadamia nuts for 2 hours.	Calories: 50, Protein: 1g, Carbs:	1 cup	5 minutes

Dairy Alternative	Ingredients	Instructions	Nutritional Information	Serving Size	Cooking Time
	water, 1 tsp vanilla extract (optional)	Drain and blend with water until smooth. Strain if desired.	1g, Fiber: 0g, Sugars: 1g, Fat: 5g, Sodium: 5mg, Potassium: 30mg		
Pea Milk	1 cup yellow split peas, 4 cups water, 1 tsp vanilla extract (optional)	Cook peas until soft. Drain and blend with water until smooth. Strain	Calories: 70, Protein: 8g, Carbs: 2g, Fiber: 1g, Sugars: 1g, Fat: 4g, Sodium:	1 cup	20 minutes

Dairy Alternative	Ingredients	Instructions	Nutritional Information	Serving Size	Cooking Time
		through a nut milk bag. Add vanilla extract if desired.	40mg, Potassium: 100mg		
Flax Milk	1/4 cup flaxseeds, 4 cups water, 1 tsp vanilla extract (optional)	Blend flaxseeds and water until smooth. Strain through a nut milk bag. Add vanilla extract if desired.	Calories: 50, Protein: 0g, Carbs: 2g, Fiber: 0g, Sugars: 1g, Fat: 5g, Sodium: 15mg, Potassium: 50mg	1 cup	5 minutes

Dairy Alternative	Ingredients	Instructions	Nutritional Information	Serving Size	Cooking Time
Hazelnut Milk	1 cup raw hazelnuts, 4 cups water, 1 tsp vanilla extract (optional)	Soak hazelnuts overnight. Drain and blend with water until smooth. Strain through a nut milk bag. Add vanilla extract if desired.	Calories: 50, Protein: 1g, Carbs: 2g, Fiber: 1g, Sugars: 1g, Fat: 5g, Sodium: 5mg, Potassium: 50mg	1 cup	10 minutes

Dairy Alternative	Ingredients	Instructions	Nutritional Information	Serving Size	Cooking Time
Quinoa Milk	1 cup cooked quinoa, 4 cups water, 1 tsp vanilla extract (optional)	Blend cooked quinoa and water until smooth. Strain through a nut milk bag. Add vanilla extract if desired.	Calories: 70, Protein: 2g, Carbs: 12g, Fiber: 1g, Sugars: 1g, Fat: 2g, Sodium: 10mg, Potassium: 80mg	1 cup	10 minutes
Pumpkin Seed Milk	1 cup raw pumpkin seeds, 4 cups water, 1	Soak pumpkin seeds for 2 hours. Drain and	Calories: 60, Protein: 3g, Carbs: 2g, Fiber:	1 cup	5 minutes

Dairy Alternative	Ingredients	Instructions	Nutritional Information	Serving Size	Cooking Time
	tsp vanilla extract (optional)	blend with water until smooth. Strain if desired. Add vanilla extract if desired.	1g, Sugars: 1g, Fat: 5g, Sodium: 10mg, Potassium: 100mg		
Sesame Seed Milk	1/2 cup sesame seeds, 4 cups water, 1 tsp vanilla extract	Blend sesame seeds and water until smooth. Strain through a nut milk	Calories: 60, Protein: 2g, Carbs: 2g, Fiber: 1g, Sugars: 0g, Fat:	1 cup	5 minutes

Dairy Alternative	Ingredients	Instructions	Nutritional Information	Serving Size	Cooking Time
	(optional)	bag. Add vanilla extract if desired.	5g, Sodium: 15mg, Potassium: 70mg		
Sunflower Seed Milk	1 cup raw sunflower seeds, 4 cups water, 1 tsp vanilla extract (optional)	Soak sunflower seeds for 2 hours. Drain and blend with water until smooth. Strain if desired. Add	Calories: 70, Protein: 2g, Carbs: 3g, Fiber: 1g, Sugars: 1g, Fat: 6g, Sodium: 10mg, Potassium: 60mg	1 cup	5 minutes

Dairy Alternative	Ingredients	Instructions	Nutritional Information	Serving Size	Cooking Time
		vanilla extract if desired.			

Snacks and Convenience Foods

Incorporating low sodium snacks and convenience foods into your diet is essential for maintaining a balanced lifestyle while managing sodium intake.

Below is a detailed table with 15 low sodium snacks and convenience foods, including ingredients, instructions, nutritional information, serving size, and cooking time.

Snack/Convenience Food	Ingredients	Instructions	Nutritional Information (per serving)	Serving Size	Cooking Time
Apple Slices with Almond Butter	1 large apple, 2 tbsp almond butter (unsalted)	Slice the apple and spread almond butter on each slice.	Calories: 200, Protein: 4g, Carbohydrates: 30g, Fiber: 5g,	1 large apple with 2 tbsp almond butter	5 minutes

Snack/Convenience Food	Ingredients	Instructions	Nutritional Information (per serving)	Serving Size	Cooking Time
			Sugars: 20g, Fat: 8g, Sodium: 0mg		
Carrot and Cucumber Sticks with Hummus	1 large carrot, 1 cucumber, 1/4 cup hummus (low sodium)	Slice carrot and cucumber into sticks, serve with hummus.	Calories: 100, Protein: 2g, Carbohydrates: 15g, Fiber: 4g, Sugars: 6g, Fat: 4g,	1 large carrot, 1 cucumber, 1/4 cup hummus	10 minutes

Snack/Convenience Food	Ingredients	Instructions	Nutritional Information (per serving)	Serving Size	Cooking Time
			Sodium: 50mg		
Greek Yogurt with Berries	1 cup plain Greek yogurt (low sodium), 1/2 cup mixed berries	Combine yogurt and berries in a bowl.	Calories: 150, Protein: 10g, Carbohydrates: 20g, Fiber: 3g, Sugars: 15g, Fat: 3g, Sodium: 60mg	1 cup yogurt with 1/2 cup berries	5 minutes

Snack/Convenience Food	Ingredients	Instructions	Nutritional Information (per serving)	Serving Size	Cooking Time
Rice Cakes with Avocado	2 plain rice cakes, 1/2 avocado, a pinch of black pepper	Mash avocado, spread on rice cakes, sprinkle with pepper.	Calories: 180, Protein: 3g, Carbohydrates: 25g, Fiber: 5g, Sugars: 0g, Fat: 10g, Sodium: 10mg	2 rice cakes with 1/2 avocado	5 minutes
Air-Popped Popcorn	3 cups air-popped popcor	Toss popcorn with olive oil	Calories: 120, Protein: 3g,	3 cups	5 minutes

Snack/Convenience Food	Ingredients	Instructions	Nutritional Information (per serving)	Serving Size	Cooking Time
	n, 1 tbsp olive oil, 1 tsp nutritional yeast	and nutritional yeast.	Carbohydrates: 18g, Fiber: 4g, Sugars: 0g, Fat: 5g, Sodium: 0mg		
Edamame	1 cup edamame (shelled), 1 tsp olive oil, a	Steam edamame, drizzle with olive oil, sprinkle	Calories: 130, Protein: 11g, Carbohydrates: 9g, Fiber:	1 cup	10 minutes

Snack/Convenience Food	Ingredients	Instructions	Nutritional Information (per serving)	Serving Size	Cooking Time
	pinch of sea salt	with salt.	4g, Sugars: 2g, Fat: 5g, Sodium: 50mg		
Celery Sticks with Cream Cheese	2 celery stalks, 2 tbsp cream cheese (low fat)	Cut celery into sticks, fill with cream cheese.	Calories: 100, Protein: 3g, Carbohydrates: 5g, Fiber: 2g, Sugars: 3g, Fat: 7g,	2 celery stalks with 2 tbsp cream chees e	5 minu tes

Snack/Convenience Food	Ingredients	Instructions	Nutritional Information (per serving)	Serving Size	Cooking Time
			Sodium: 75mg		
Cottage Cheese with Pineapple	1/2 cup cottage cheese (low sodium), 1/2 cup pineapple chunks	Mix cottage cheese and pineapple chunks in a bowl.	Calories: 140, Protein: 12g, Carbohydrates: 15g, Fiber: 1g, Sugars: 13g, Fat: 3g, Sodium: 150mg	1/2 cup cottage cheese with 1/2 cup pineapple	5 minutes

Snack/Convenience Food	Ingredients	Instructions	Nutritional Information (per serving)	Serving Size	Cooking Time
Cherry Tomatoes with Mozzarella	1 cup cherry tomatoes, 1/2 cup mozzarella balls (low sodium)	Combine cherry tomatoes and mozzarella balls in a bowl.	Calories: 150, Protein: 10g, Carbohydrates: 7g, Fiber: 2g, Sugars: 5g, Fat: 10g, Sodium: 100mg	1 cup tomatoes with 1/2 cup mozzarella	5 minutes

Snack/Convenience Food	Ingredients	Instructions	Nutritional Information (per serving)	Serving Size	Cooking Time
Almonds and Raisins Mix	1/4 cup unsalted almonds, 1/4 cup raisins	Mix almonds and raisins together in a bowl.	Calories: 200, Protein: 6g, Carbohydrates: 28g, Fiber: 4g, Sugars: 18g, Fat: 10g, Sodium: 0mg	1/2 cup mix	2 minutes

Snack/Convenience Food	Ingredients	Instructions	Nutritional Information (per serving)	Serving Size	Cooking Time
Baked Sweet Potato Chips	1 large sweet potato, 1 tbsp olive oil, a pinch of paprika	Slice sweet potato thinly, toss with olive oil and paprika, bake at 400°F for 20 minutes.	Calories: 160, Protein: 2g, Carbohydrates: 28g, Fiber: 4g, Sugars: 8g, Fat: 6g, Sodium: 30mg	1 large sweet potato	25 minutes

Snack/Convenience Food	Ingredients	Instructions	Nutritional Information (per serving)	Serving Size	Cooking Time
Oatmeal with Banana and Cinnamon	1/2 cup rolled oats, 1 cup water, 1/2 banana, 1/4 tsp cinnamon	Cook oats with water, slice banana, top oatmeal with banana and cinnamon.	Calories: 200, Protein: 5g, Carbohydrates: 40g, Fiber: 5g, Sugars: 12g, Fat: 3g, Sodium: 0mg	1 bowl	10 minutes

Snack/Convenience Food	Ingredients	Instructions	Nutritional Information (per serving)	Serving Size	Cooking Time
Sliced Bell Peppers with Guacamole	1 bell pepper, 1/4 cup guacamole	Slice bell pepper, serve with guacamole.	Calories: 150, Protein: 2g, Carbohydrates: 10g, Fiber: 5g, Sugars: 4g, Fat: 10g, Sodium: 100mg	1 bell pepper with 1/4 cup guacamole	5 minutes
Yogurt with Honey and Walnuts	1 cup plain Greek yogurt,	Mix yogurt with honey,	Calories: 200, Protein: 10g,	1 cup yogurt with	5 minutes

Snack/Convenience Food	Ingredients	Instructions	Nutritional Information (per serving)	Serving Size	Cooking Time
	1 tbsp honey, 2 tbsp walnuts (unsalted)	top with walnuts.	Carbohydrates: 20g, Fiber: 2g, Sugars: 18g, Fat: 8g, Sodium: 50mg	toppings	

Snack/Convenience Food	Ingredients	Instructions	Nutritional Information (per serving)	Serving Size	Cooking Time
Turkey and Avocado Roll-Ups	4 slices turkey breast (low sodium), 1/2 avocado, 1 tsp lemon juice	Mash avocado with lemon juice, spread on turkey slices, roll up.	Calories: 150, Protein: 15g, Carbohydrates: 5g, Fiber: 3g, Sugars: 0g, Fat: 8g, Sodium: 200mg	4 roll-ups	5 minutes

These low sodium snacks and convenience foods provide a variety of options to help you maintain a balanced and enjoyable diet while managing your sodium intake.

Chapter 5: Foods to Avoid

Processed and Packaged Foods

Processed and packaged foods often contain high levels of sodium, which can be detrimental to your health, especially if you are following a low sodium diet.

These foods typically have added salt for preservation and flavor enhancement. Excessive sodium intake is linked to high blood pressure, heart disease, and other health issues.

Below is a detailed table outlining various processed and packaged foods you should avoid and the reasons why they should be excluded from your diet.

Processed and Packaged Food	Examples	Reasons to Avoid
Canned Soups and Stews	Chicken noodle soup, beef stew, vegetable soup	These products are often loaded with sodium to enhance flavor and preserve shelf life. A single serving can contain more than half of the

Processed and Packaged Food	Examples	Reasons to Avoid
		recommended daily sodium intake, making it easy to exceed your daily limit.
Processed Meats	Bacon, sausage, hot dogs, deli meats	Processed meats are high in sodium due to curing, smoking, and seasoning processes. Consuming these regularly can lead to increased blood pressure and a higher risk of cardiovascular diseases.
Frozen Dinners	Pizza, lasagna, pot pies, TV dinners	Frozen meals are convenient but notoriously high in sodium to maintain flavor and extend shelf life. They can contain upwards of 1,000 mg of sodium

Processed and Packaged Food	Examples	Reasons to Avoid
		per serving, which is nearly half the daily recommended amount.
Snack Foods	Potato chips, pretzels, salted nuts, popcorn	These snacks are typically coated in salt for flavor. Regular consumption can easily lead to excessive sodium intake, contributing to high blood pressure and other health issues.
Condiments and Sauces	Soy sauce, ketchup, salad dressings, barbecue sauce	Many condiments are high in sodium to enhance taste. A single tablespoon of soy sauce, for example, can contain around 1,000 mg of sodium. Using these regularly

Processed and Packaged Food	Examples	Reasons to Avoid
		can quickly add up to a high sodium intake.
Instant Noodles	Ramen, cup noodles, instant pasta	Instant noodles come with flavor packets that are extremely high in sodium. A single serving can often exceed the daily recommended sodium intake, making it easy to overconsume.
Packaged Snacks and Crackers	Cheese crackers, salted rice cakes, flavored nuts	These snacks are convenient but often high in sodium to enhance their taste and preserve freshness. Consuming them regularly can contribute to an unhealthy sodium intake.

Processed and Packaged Food	Examples	Reasons to Avoid
Canned Vegetables and Beans	Canned green beans, corn, baked beans	While vegetables are healthy, the canned versions often have added salt for preservation. Opting for fresh or frozen vegetables without added salt is a better alternative.
Ready-to-Eat Breakfast Cereals	Flavored oatmeals, pre-sweetened cereals	Many ready-to-eat cereals contain added sodium as a preservative and flavor enhancer. Choosing plain, unsweetened cereals can help reduce sodium intake.
Packaged Breads and Bakery Products	White bread, muffins, bagels	Packaged bakery products often contain high levels of sodium. Even

Processed and Packaged Food	Examples	Reasons to Avoid
		seemingly healthy options like whole grain bread can have significant amounts of added salt.
Cheese and Dairy Products	Processed cheese slices, cheese spreads, flavored yogurts	Processed cheeses and some flavored dairy products contain high levels of sodium. Choosing low sodium or fresh cheese and plain dairy products is a healthier option.
Packaged Condiments	Pickles, olives, relish	Packaged condiments are preserved in salty brines, making them high in sodium. These should be consumed sparingly to avoid excessive sodium intake.

Processed and Packaged Food	Examples	Reasons to Avoid
Fast Food and Restaurant Meals	Burgers, fries, pizza, Chinese takeout	Fast food and restaurant meals are often loaded with sodium to enhance flavor and preserve ingredients. Opting for homemade meals or requesting no added salt can help reduce sodium intake.
Microwaveable Meals	Microwaveable burritos, mac and cheese, ready-to-eat meals	These meals are convenient but typically high in sodium. Preparing fresh meals at home allows better control over sodium content.
Salty Snacks	Beef jerky, pork rinds, salted crackers	Salty snacks are popular for their taste but are very high in sodium. Consuming these regularly can

Processed and Packaged Food	Examples	Reasons to Avoid
		contribute to high blood pressure and other sodium-related health issues.

Avoiding this high sodium processed and packaged foods is essential for maintaining a low sodium diet and improving your overall health.

By focusing on fresh, whole foods and preparing meals at home, you can better control your sodium intake and support a healthier lifestyle.

Snacks and Junk Food

Avoiding high sodium snacks and junk food is crucial for maintaining a healthy diet and managing sodium intake.

The following table outlines common high sodium snacks and junk foods, explaining why they should be avoided as part of a low sodium lifestyle.

Snack/Junk Food	Description	Sodium Content	Reasons to Avoid
Potato Chips	Thinly sliced, deep-fried, and often heavily salted.	High, often 200-300mg per serving.	Excessive sodium contributes to high blood pressure and increases the risk of heart disease.
Pretzels	Baked dough snacks, often salted.	High, around 400-500mg per serving.	High sodium content can lead to water retention and elevated blood pressure.

Snack/Junk Food	Description	Sodium Content	Reasons to Avoid
Salted Nuts	Nuts roasted and salted, such as peanuts or cashews.	High, varying from 100-250mg per serving.	Sodium masks the natural health benefits of nuts, such as heart-healthy fats and protein.
Microwave Popcorn	Pre-packaged popcorn often with added butter and salt.	Very high, up to 600mg per bag.	Contains high levels of sodium and often unhealthy trans fats.
Processed Cheese Snacks	Cheese-flavored snacks, like cheese puffs and crackers.	High, around 250-400mg per serving.	High sodium and unhealthy additives increase health risks.
Beef Jerky	Dried, seasoned meat, often highly salted	Very high, around 500-700m	Excessive sodium intake can harm kidney function

Snack/Junk Food	Description	Sodium Content	Reasons to Avoid
	for preservation.	g per serving.	and elevate blood pressure.
Instant Noodles	Pre-packaged noodles with seasoning packets.	Extremely high, often over 1000mg per serving.	High in sodium and unhealthy additives, contributing to hypertension and heart issues.
Canned Soups	Ready-to-eat soups often high in sodium for flavor and preservation.	Very high, around 700-900mg per serving.	High sodium content can lead to high blood pressure and increased cardiovascular risk.
Frozen Dinners	Pre-cooked meals that are reheated in the microwave.	High, around 500-800mg per meal.	High sodium content and preservatives negatively

Snack/Junk Food	Description	Sodium Content	Reasons to Avoid
			impact heart health.
Pizza	Especially frozen or restaurant pizza, often with salty toppings.	Extremely high, 600-1000 mg per slice.	Combines high sodium with unhealthy fats, increasing heart disease risk.
French Fries	Deep-fried potatoes, often heavily salted.	High, around 300-400mg per serving.	High sodium and unhealthy fats contribute to heart disease and hypertension.
Sausages and Hot Dogs	Processed meats, often preserved with sodium.	Very high, 500-800mg per item.	Linked to increased risk of heart disease and high blood pressure.

Snack/Junk Food	Description	Sodium Content	Reasons to Avoid
Breaded Chicken Tenders	Chicken coated in breadcrumbs and fried, often salted.	High, around 500-600mg per serving.	High sodium and unhealthy fats contribute to poor cardiovascular health.
Flavored Crackers	Crackers with added seasonings, often salty.	High, around 250-400mg per serving.	High sodium content can lead to elevated blood pressure and heart issues.
Pickles	Cucumbers preserved in brine, heavily salted.	Very high, around 700-900mg per serving.	High sodium content can lead to water retention and hypertension.

These high sodium snacks and junk foods contribute to excessive sodium intake, which can lead to a range of health issues, including high blood pressure, heart disease, and kidney problems.

Avoiding these foods and opting for low sodium alternatives is a key step in maintaining a healthy and balanced diet.

Condiments and Sauces

Condiments and sauces often contain high levels of sodium, which can contribute significantly to your daily sodium intake. For individuals following a low sodium diet, it's essential to be mindful of these hidden sources of sodium.

Below is a detailed table that includes common condiments and sauces to avoid, along with explanations of why they should be avoided.

Condiment/Sauce	Reason to Avoid	Typical Sodium Content (per serving)
Soy Sauce	Soy sauce is extremely high in sodium, with just one tablespoon containing a significant portion of the recommended daily sodium intake. This can	Approximately 920 mg per tablespoon

Condiment/Sauce	Reason to Avoid	Typical Sodium Content (per serving)
	quickly add up, especially if used frequently in cooking or as a table condiment.	
Ketchup	Ketchup contains added salt and often high amounts of sugar. Although it is used in small quantities, frequent use can lead to excessive sodium consumption.	Approximately 160 mg per tablespoon
Barbecue Sauce	Barbecue sauce is typically high in sodium and sugar, making it a	Approximately 300 mg per 2 tablespoons

Condiment/Sauce	Reason to Avoid	Typical Sodium Content (per serving)
	double threat for those on low sodium diets. It is often used in larger quantities, which can increase sodium intake substantially.	
Salad Dressings	Many commercial salad dressings contain high levels of sodium to enhance flavor and preserve the product. Creamy dressings, in particular, can be	Approximately 300 mg per 2 tablespoons

Condiment/Sauce	Reason to Avoid	Typical Sodium Content (per serving)
	quite high in sodium.	
Teriyaki Sauce	Teriyaki sauce is similar to soy sauce in its high sodium content. It is often used as a marinade or glaze, adding significant sodium to meals.	Approximately 600 mg per tablespoon
Mustard	Although mustard may seem innocuous, it can contain high levels of sodium. It is commonly used in sandwiches and as a	Approximately 120 mg per teaspoon

Condiment/Sauce	Reason to Avoid	Typical Sodium Content (per serving)
	condiment, adding to daily sodium intake.	
Hot Sauce	Hot sauces vary widely in sodium content, but many are high in sodium due to the added salt for preservation and flavor. Frequent use can contribute to excessive sodium intake.	Approximately 200 mg per teaspoon
Marinara Sauce	Store-bought marinara sauce can be high in sodium, often due to added salt	Approximately 480 mg per 1/2 cup

Condiment/Sauce	Reason to Avoid	Typical Sodium Content (per serving)
	for flavor enhancement and preservation. It is typically used in pasta dishes and can add up quickly.	
Pickles	Pickles are preserved in a brine solution, which is high in salt. Eating pickles regularly can lead to high sodium consumption, making them a food to avoid on a low sodium diet.	Approximately 350 mg per medium pickle

Condiment/Sauce	Reason to Avoid	Typical Sodium Content (per serving)
Soy-based Condiments (e.g., Hoisin Sauce, Miso)	These condiments, like soy sauce, are high in sodium. They are used in various Asian dishes and can significantly increase sodium intake when used regularly.	Hoisin Sauce: Approximately 500 mg per tablespoon; Miso: Approximately 630 mg per tablespoon
Relish	Relish, particularly sweet pickle relish, contains added salt and sugar. It is commonly used in sandwiches and salads,	Approximately 180 mg per tablespoon

Condiment/Sauce	Reason to Avoid	Typical Sodium Content (per serving)
	contributing to overall sodium intake.	
Worcestershire Sauce	Worcestershire sauce contains a variety of ingredients, including salt, that contribute to its high sodium content. It is often used in marinades and sauces, adding to sodium intake.	Approximately 65 mg per teaspoon
Ranch Dressing	Ranch dressing is a popular condiment that is high in sodium and fat. It is	Approximately 320 mg per 2 tablespoons

Condiment/Sauce	Reason to Avoid	Typical Sodium Content (per serving)
	often used in salads and as a dip, which can lead to high sodium consumption.	
Tartar Sauce	Tartar sauce, often used with seafood, contains added salt and can be high in sodium. Regular use can contribute to excessive sodium intake.	Approximately 190 mg per tablespoon
Steak Sauce	Steak sauce contains a variety of sodium-rich ingredients. It is	Approximately 280 mg per tablespoon

Condiment/Sauce	Reason to Avoid	Typical Sodium Content (per serving)
	used as a condiment for meats, adding substantial sodium to meals.	

Avoiding these high-sodium condiments and sauces can help you better manage your sodium intake and support a healthier diet.

Option for homemade versions or low sodium alternatives whenever possible to maintain flavor without compromising your health goals.

Baked Goods

Baked goods are a popular and convenient food category, but many of these items contain high levels of sodium, which can be detrimental to your health, especially if you are following a low sodium diet.

Here is a comprehensive table detailing various baked goods that you should avoid, along with explanations of why they are not suitable for a low sodium diet.

Baked Goods	Reasons to Avoid	Sodium Content	Alternative Options
White Bread	White bread often contains added salt to enhance flavor and preserve freshness. Consuming it regularly can significantly increase your	Approximately 150-200 mg per slice	Opt for homemade bread using low sodium recipes or buy low sodium whole grain bread.

Baked Goods	Reasons to Avoid	Sodium Content	Alternative Options
	sodium intake.		
Bagels	Bagels are typically high in sodium due to the ingredients used in the dough and the salt added on top.	Approximately 400-500 mg per bagel	Choose low sodium bagels or make your own using a low sodium recipe.
Biscuits	Biscuits often contain high amounts of sodium from both baking powder and salt added for flavor.	Approximately 300-400 mg per biscuit	Make homemade biscuits with low sodium baking powder and no added salt.

Baked Goods	Reasons to Avoid	Sodium Content	Alternative Options
Croissants	Croissants are high in sodium due to the salted butter and additional salt used in the dough.	Approximately 350-450 mg per croissant	Consider making low sodium versions at home or choose whole grain alternatives.
Muffins	Store-bought muffins often have high sodium levels due to the ingredients and preservatives used.	Approximately 300-400 mg per muffin	Make homemade muffins using fresh ingredients and low sodium baking powder.
Pretzels	Pretzels are known for their high salt content, both in the dough	Approximately 400-600 mg per serving	Opt for unsalted pretzels or make your own

Baked Goods	Reasons to Avoid	Sodium Content	Alternative Options
	and on the surface.		using a low sodium recipe.
Pizza Crust	Store-bought pizza crusts are usually high in sodium due to added salt and preservatives.	Approximately 400-600 mg per slice	Make homemade pizza dough with minimal salt or buy low sodium crust options.
Cookies	Packaged cookies often contain high levels of sodium due to preservatives and added salt for flavor.	Approximately 100-200 mg per cookie	Bake homemade cookies using low sodium recipes and natural ingredients.

Baked Goods	Reasons to Avoid	Sodium Content	Alternative Options
Cake Mixes	Commercial cake mixes include high sodium levels from baking powder and preservatives.	Approximately 300-400 mg per slice	Prepare cakes from scratch using low sodium baking powder and fresh ingredients.
Pie Crusts	Pre-made pie crusts are typically high in sodium from the shortening and added salt.	Approximately 200-300 mg per slice	Make pie crusts at home with unsalted butter and no added salt.
Scones	Scones often contain significant amounts of sodium from baking	Approximately 300-400 mg per scone	Use low sodium baking powder and unsalted butter to make homemade scones.

Baked Goods	Reasons to Avoid	Sodium Content	Alternative Options
	powder and added salt.		
Crackers	Many commercial crackers have high sodium levels due to added salt and preservatives.	Approximately 200-300 mg per serving	Choose unsalted or low sodium crackers, or make your own at home.
Tortillas	Store-bought tortillas can be high in sodium due to preservatives and added salt.	Approximately 200-300 mg per tortilla	Make homemade tortillas using low sodium recipes or buy low sodium options.
Donuts	Donuts contain high sodium levels from both	Approximately 200-300 mg per donut	Opt for homemade donuts with minimal added

Baked Goods	Reasons to Avoid	Sodium Content	Alternative Options
	the dough and the icing/glaze.		salt or choose low sodium recipes.
Pancakes	Pancake mixes and restaurant pancakes often have high sodium from baking powder and added salt.	Approximately 200-300 mg per pancake	Make pancakes from scratch using low sodium baking powder and fresh ingredients.

Avoiding high sodium baked goods is essential for maintaining a low sodium diet and supporting overall health.

By being aware of the sodium content in these common items and opting for homemade or low sodium alternatives, you can significantly reduce your sodium intake.

Incorporate fresh ingredients and low sodium baking methods to enjoy baked goods without compromising your health goals.

Chapter 6: Low Sodium Meal Planning

Weekly Meal Planning Tips

Weekly meal planning is a crucial strategy for maintaining a low sodium diet and ensuring you consistently consume healthy, balanced meals. Start by setting aside time each week to plan your meals.

Consider your schedule, including busy days when you might need quicker options, and more relaxed days when you can prepare more elaborate dishes. By organizing your meals in advance, you reduce the temptation to reach for high sodium convenience foods.

Begin your meal planning by reviewing the Low Sodium Food List 2024. This list will guide you in selecting ingredients that are naturally low in sodium, such as fresh fruits, vegetables, lean proteins, and whole grains.

 Incorporate a variety of these foods to create diverse and satisfying meals. Variety is key to preventing boredom and ensuring you get a broad range of nutrients.

Once you have a list of low sodium foods, start mapping out your meals for the week. Plan for breakfast, lunch, dinner, and snacks, ensuring each meal is balanced and adheres to your sodium intake goals.

Think about incorporating different cooking methods, such as grilling, baking, steaming, and sautéing, to keep your meals interesting and flavorful. Remember to include fresh herbs and spices as sodium-free flavor enhancers.

Creating a detailed grocery list is an essential part of the meal planning process. List all the ingredients you need for the week based on your meal plan.

Sticking to this list while shopping helps you avoid impulse purchases of high sodium foods. If possible, shop the perimeter of the grocery store where fresh produce, meats, and dairy are typically located, and limit time spent in aisles with processed foods.

Meal prep can save you time during the week and help ensure you stick to your low sodium diet. Set aside a few hours after grocery shopping to prepare ingredients or even cook complete meals.
Chop vegetables, cook grains, and portion out snacks in advance. Store these prepared items in airtight containers so they are ready to

use when you need them. This approach minimizes the effort required to put together a healthy meal during busy weekdays.

It's important to be flexible with your meal plan. Life can be unpredictable, and there may be days when your schedule changes. Having a few backup meals or snacks prepared can help you stay on track.

Keep easy-to-make, low sodium options in your pantry or freezer for such occasions. This way, you can adapt to changes without compromising your dietary goals.

Incorporating these weekly meal planning tips into your routine can make a significant difference in managing your sodium intake and overall health.

By consistently planning, shopping, and preparing low sodium meals, you create a sustainable habit that supports your long-term wellness. Use the Low Sodium Food List 2024 as your guide and embrace the process of planning and preparing meals that nourish your body and fit your lifestyle.

Creating Balanced, Low Sodium Meals

Creating balanced, low sodium meals is essential for maintaining your health and well-being, particularly if you're managing conditions like hypertension or kidney disease. The first step is to plan your meals around fresh, whole foods that are naturally low in sodium.

Fruits and vegetables should be the cornerstone of your diet, providing essential vitamins, minerals, and fiber without the added sodium found in many processed foods. Option
for fresh produce over canned or frozen varieties, unless they are labeled "no salt added."

Lean proteins are another critical component of a balanced, low sodium meal. Fresh poultry, fish, and lean cuts of meat are excellent choices. Avoid processed meats like deli cuts, bacon, and sausages, which are often high in sodium.

When preparing meat, use herbs, spices, and citrus juices for seasoning instead of salt. This not only enhances the flavor but also helps you stay within your sodium limits.

Whole grains should also be included in your meal planning. Foods like brown rice, quinoa, and whole wheat pasta are nutritious and naturally low in sodium.

When choosing bread, cereals, or other grain-based products, look for those labeled "low sodium" or "no salt added." Cooking grains at home gives you control over the ingredients, allowing you to avoid hidden sodium often found in pre-packaged varieties.

Dairy products can be a hidden source of sodium, so it's important to select low sodium options. Choose plain yogurt, milk, and cheeses that are labeled low sodium or no sodium.

Be mindful of portion sizes with dairy products, as even low sodium varieties can add up if consumed in large quantities. Incorporating unsweetened almond milk or other dairy alternatives can also help reduce your sodium intake.

Legumes and nuts are excellent additions to a low sodium diet, providing protein, fiber, and healthy fats. Opt for unsalted varieties of nuts and seeds, and use dried beans or no-salt-added canned beans in your recipes.

Legumes can be used in salads, soups, and stews to add texture and nutrition without the added sodium.

Cooking methods play a significant role in maintaining a low sodium diet. Grilling, steaming, roasting, and baking are all excellent techniques that can bring out the natural flavors of food without the need for added salt.

Using fresh herbs, garlic, onions, and lemon juice can enhance the taste of your meals. Experimenting with different spice blends and seasoning mixes can also provide a flavorful alternative to salt.

Finally, meal planning and preparation are crucial for maintaining a balanced, low sodium diet. Set aside time each week to plan your meals, create a shopping list, and prepare ingredients in advance.

This not only ensures that you have healthy, low sodium options readily available but also helps you avoid the temptation of high sodium convenience foods.

By staying organized and committed to your meal plan, you can enjoy delicious, nutritious meals that support your health and well-being.

Grocery Shopping Strategies

Grocery shopping for a low sodium diet requires careful planning and informed choices. Begin by creating a detailed shopping list before heading to the store.

This list should include fresh fruits and vegetables, lean meats, whole grains, and other low sodium staples. By sticking to your list, you can avoid impulse purchases of high sodium items and ensure you have all the ingredients needed for your meal plan.

When selecting produce, choose fresh fruits and vegetables, as they are naturally low in sodium. Option for a variety of colors and types to ensure a range of nutrients. If fresh produce is not available, frozen vegetables without added sauces or seasonings are a great alternative.

Canned vegetables can also be used, but be sure to choose those labeled "no salt added" and rinse them thoroughly to reduce sodium content.

For protein sources, focus on fresh, unprocessed meats, poultry, and fish. Avoid pre-marinated or pre-seasoned options, as these often contain high levels of sodium.

If you prefer plant-based proteins, include legumes, beans, and tofu in your shopping list. When buying canned beans, select low sodium versions and rinse them before use to remove excess sodium.

Whole grains are an essential part of a low sodium diet. Choose plain whole grains like brown rice, quinoa, and whole wheat pasta. Avoid instant or flavored grain products, which typically contain added sodium. Incorporate a variety of grains into your meals to keep them interesting and nutritionally balanced.

Dairy products can be tricky, as many cheeses and processed dairy items are high in sodium. Option for low sodium or sodium-free versions of cheese, yogurt, and milk.

If you're unsure about the sodium content, always check the nutrition label. Unsweetened plant-based milks, like almond or oat milk, can also be good alternatives with lower sodium levels.

Processed and packaged foods are major sources of hidden sodium, so it's crucial to read nutrition labels carefully.

Look for items labeled "low sodium," "reduced sodium," or "no salt added." Be cautious with terms like "reduced sodium," which means the product contains at least 25% less sodium than the regular version but may still be high in sodium.

Aim for products with 5% or less of the daily value for sodium per serving.

Lastly, shop the perimeter of the grocery store, where fresh produce, meats, and dairy are typically located. The inner aisles often contain processed and packaged foods that are high in sodium.

By focusing on fresh, whole foods and being diligent about reading labels, you can effectively manage your sodium intake and support your overall health. This strategic approach to grocery shopping, combined with a well-planned meal strategy, will help you maintain a successful low sodium lifestyle.

Chapter 7: Cooking Techniques

Using Fresh Herbs and Spices

Using fresh herbs and spices is an excellent way to enhance the flavor of your dishes while adhering to a low sodium diet. These natural flavor enhancers can transform your meals, making them more enjoyable without the need for added salt.

Fresh herbs like basil, cilantro, parsley, and thyme offer a burst of freshness and aroma that can elevate any dish, from salads to soups and main courses.

Spices such as cumin, turmeric, paprika, and cinnamon add depth and complexity, providing a rich, savory, or sweet profile depending on the dish.

Incorporating fresh herbs into your cooking involves understanding the best times to add them to your dishes.

Delicate herbs like basil, parsley, and cilantro are best added towards the end of the cooking process or used as a garnish to preserve their vibrant flavor and color.

Heartier herbs like rosemary and thyme can be added earlier during cooking to allow their flavors to meld with the dish. Experimenting with different combinations of herbs can lead to discovering new and exciting flavor profiles that satisfy your taste buds without the need for excess sodium.

Spices, on the other hand, can be used at various stages of cooking to build layers of flavor. Toasting whole spices like cumin seeds, coriander seeds, and mustard seeds in a dry pan before grinding them can intensify their flavors.

Ground spices can be added at the beginning of cooking to infuse the oil with their essence, or towards the end for a more pronounced taste.

Balancing the use of spices with fresh herbs can create a well-rounded flavor profile that enhances your culinary creations while keeping sodium levels in check.

Growing your own herbs can be a rewarding and cost-effective way to ensure you always have fresh ingredients on hand. Herbs like basil, mint, and oregano can be grown in small pots on a windowsill or in a garden.

This not only provides a fresh supply of herbs but also allows you to control the quality and ensure they are free from pesticides and other contaminants. Using homegrown herbs in your cooking can also enhance the satisfaction of preparing and enjoying meals that are both healthy and flavorful.

When substituting fresh herbs and spices for salt, it's important to understand the potency and balance required to achieve the desired flavor.

For instance, a combination of garlic, lemon zest, and parsley can provide a bright and zesty flavor that complements fish or chicken dishes. Similarly, using a blend of cumin, coriander, and paprika can create a rich and smoky flavor ideal for grilled meats and vegetables.

The key is to experiment with different combinations and quantities to find what works best for your palate and the specific dish you are preparing.

To maximize the flavor of herbs and spices, consider using them in marinades, dressings, and rubs. Marinating proteins like chicken, fish, or tofu in a mixture of herbs, spices, olive oil, and a splash of vinegar or citrus juice can infuse the food with intense flavors while keeping it moist and tender.

Homemade dressings made with fresh herbs, garlic, lemon juice, and a bit of olive oil can transform salads into vibrant, flavorful meals. Spice rubs can be used to coat meats and vegetables before grilling or roasting, creating a flavorful crust that enhances the overall taste.

Ultimately, using fresh herbs and spices is a versatile and healthy way to add flavor to your meals without relying on sodium.

By experimenting with different herbs and spice combinations, growing your own herbs, and incorporating these ingredients at various stages of cooking, you can create delicious, low-sodium dishes that are satisfying and nutritious.

Embracing the use of fresh herbs and spices in your cooking not only supports your low sodium lifestyle but also opens up a world of culinary possibilities that keep your meals exciting and full of flavor.

Flavor Enhancers Without Sodium

Enhancing the flavor of your food without relying on sodium can be a game-changer for maintaining a low sodium diet. One of the most effective ways to achieve this is by using fresh herbs.

Basil, cilantro, parsley, and dill can add vibrant, aromatic notes to your dishes. Incorporating these herbs not only enhances flavor but also adds a nutritional boost. For example, basil can transform a simple tomato salad, while cilantro can elevate the taste of a homemade salsa.

Spices are another excellent way to enhance flavor without adding sodium. Cumin, paprika, turmeric, and cinnamon can provide depth and complexity to your meals.

A sprinkle of smoked paprika can add a rich, smoky flavor to roasted vegetables or grilled chicken, while turmeric can lend a warm, earthy taste to soups and stews. Experimenting with different spice combinations can lead to delightful new flavor profiles that make your meals more exciting.

Citrus fruits such as lemons, limes, and oranges are fantastic for adding a tangy brightness to your dishes.

A squeeze of lemon juice can bring out the flavors in a dish of steamed vegetables or a piece of grilled fish. Lime juice can add a zesty kick to a salad or a marinade for poultry.

Orange zest can be used to infuse baked goods with a refreshing citrus note. The acidity of citrus fruits can help balance flavors and reduce the need for added salt.

Vinegars are versatile flavor enhancers that come in many varieties, each with its unique taste. Balsamic vinegar adds a sweet, tangy richness to salads, while apple cider vinegar can bring a subtle tartness to coleslaw or braised dishes.

Red wine vinegar and rice vinegar are also great for marinating meats and making dressings. Using vinegars can help you achieve complex flavors without relying on sodium.

Garlic and onions are staple ingredients that can add a robust, savory depth to your cooking. Sautéing garlic in olive oil releases its natural sugars and creates a sweet, aromatic base for many dishes.

Caramelized onions can add a sweet and savory flavor to soups, stews, and sandwiches.

Roasted garlic, with its mellow and slightly sweet taste, can be used as a spread or added to mashed potatoes for a flavorful twist.

Using umami-rich ingredients like mushrooms, tomatoes, and aged cheeses in moderation can also enhance flavor without excessive sodium.

Mushrooms, especially varieties like shiitake or portobello, have a naturally savory taste that can enrich soups, stir-fries, and sauces. Sun-dried tomatoes can add a concentrated burst of flavor to pastas and salads.

A small amount of Parmesan cheese can be used to finish a dish, adding a nutty and savory note without overloading it with sodium.

Finally, consider using homemade broths and stocks instead of store-bought versions, which can be high in sodium. Making your own broth allows you to control the ingredients and sodium content.

Simmering bones, vegetables, and herbs for several hours can create a rich, flavorful base for soups, stews, and sauces. By relying on natural flavor enhancers and cooking techniques, you can create delicious, satisfying meals that support your low sodium lifestyle.

Cooking Methods That Preserve Flavor

Cooking methods that preserve flavor while adhering to a low sodium diet are essential for maintaining a satisfying and healthy eating routine.

By focusing on techniques that enhance the natural flavors of food, you can reduce the need for added salt without sacrificing taste. Understanding these methods allows you to create delicious meals that align with your dietary goals.

One effective approach is to use fresh herbs and spices. Ingredients like garlic, ginger, basil, rosemary, thyme, and cilantro can add depth and complexity to your dishes. Experimenting with different combinations of herbs and spices can transform simple ingredients into flavorful masterpieces.

For example, marinating chicken in a mix of garlic, lemon juice, and fresh rosemary before grilling can produce a savory and aromatic dish that requires no added salt.

Roasting is another excellent method for enhancing flavor without relying on sodium.

Roasting vegetables, meats, and even fruits at high temperatures caramelizes their natural sugars, creating a rich, sweet, and savory taste. Vegetables like carrots, bell peppers, and Brussels sprouts develop a delightful sweetness when roasted, while meats gain a deliciously crispy exterior and juicy interior.

Adding a drizzle of olive oil and a sprinkle of black pepper or paprika can further elevate the flavors.

Sautéing and stir-frying are quick cooking methods that can help preserve the texture and taste of your ingredients. Using a small amount of healthy oil, such as olive or avocado oil, and cooking over medium-high heat allows the ingredients to cook quickly, locking in their natural flavors.

Incorporating aromatic vegetables like onions, garlic, and bell peppers, along with low sodium soy sauce or a splash of vinegar, can create vibrant and flavorful dishes.

Steaming is a gentle cooking method that helps retain the nutrients and natural flavors of vegetables, fish, and poultry. By steaming, you avoid the need for added fats and sodium.

Steamed vegetables can be brightened with a squeeze of lemon juice or a dash of balsamic vinegar, while steamed fish can be enhanced with fresh herbs and a hint of garlic. This method is ideal for maintaining the integrity of delicate ingredients while ensuring they remain tender and flavorful.

Slow cooking and braising are techniques that involve cooking ingredients slowly over low heat, allowing flavors to meld and intensify. These methods are perfect for tougher cuts of meat and hearty vegetables, transforming them into tender, flavorful dishes.

Using low sodium broths or homemade stocks, along with a variety of herbs and spices, can result in rich and satisfying meals without the need for added salt. The slow cooking process allows the ingredients to absorb the flavors, creating a depth of taste that is both comforting and delicious.

Grilling is a popular method that imparts a smoky, charred flavor to meats, vegetables, and even fruits. The high heat of the grill sears the exterior, locking in juices and enhancing the natural taste of the ingredients.

Marinating foods in a mixture of olive oil, vinegar, and herbs before grilling can add an extra layer of flavor. Grilled vegetables like zucchini, eggplant, and corn can be particularly delightful, offering a robust and satisfying taste without the need for salt.

Incorporating these cooking techniques into your culinary repertoire can help you create flavorful, low sodium meals that are both nutritious and enjoyable.

By emphasizing the natural tastes of your ingredients and using herbs, spices, and healthy cooking methods, you can maintain a satisfying diet without relying on added sodium. These strategies not only support your health goals but also ensure that your meals remain exciting and full of flavor.

Chapter 8: Sample Meal Plans

7Day Low Sodium Meal Plan

Creating a 7-day low sodium meal plan can help you maintain a healthy diet while managing your sodium intake effectively. Start each day with a nutritious breakfast that includes options like oatmeal with fresh fruits, Greek yogurt with berries, or a vegetable omelet.

These choices provide a balanced mix of protein, fiber, and essential vitamins while keeping sodium levels in check. It's important to use herbs and spices instead of salt to enhance the flavor of your morning meals.

Lunches can be delicious and varied with dishes such as grilled chicken salads, quinoa bowls with roasted vegetables, or turkey and avocado wraps. Using fresh, unprocessed ingredients helps keep sodium levels low.

Prepare dressings and sauces at home to control the amount of salt added, and opt for low sodium condiments. Incorporating a variety of colorful vegetables and lean proteins ensures that your meals are both satisfying and nutrient-dense.

For dinner, focus on simple yet flavorful dishes like baked salmon with a side of steamed broccoli, stir-fried tofu with mixed vegetables, or a hearty lentil soup.

Cooking at home allows you to control the sodium content and experiment with different herbs, spices, and cooking techniques. Baking, grilling, and steaming are great methods to preserve the natural flavors of your ingredients without needing to add much salt.

Snacks are an important part of a low sodium diet and can include fresh fruit, unsalted nuts, and homemade hummus with veggie sticks. These options provide essential nutrients and keep you satisfied between meals.

It's beneficial to prepare snacks in advance to avoid reaching for high sodium convenience foods. Keeping healthy snacks readily available can help maintain your energy levels throughout the day.

Planning your meals for the entire week can help streamline your shopping and preparation process. Create a detailed grocery list based on your meal plan, focusing on fresh produce, lean proteins, whole grains, and low sodium alternatives.

Batch cooking and meal prepping can save time and ensure you always have healthy options on hand, reducing the temptation to opt for high sodium convenience foods.

Hydration is also crucial in a low sodium diet. Drink plenty of water throughout the day to help flush excess sodium from your body. Herbal teas and infused water with fresh fruits and herbs are great alternatives to sugary and high sodium beverages.

Limiting the intake of processed drinks and focusing on natural, low sodium options will support your overall health and hydration.

By following a 7-day low sodium meal plan, you can effectively manage your sodium intake while enjoying a variety of delicious and nutritious meals. This approach not only supports your health goals but also encourages creativity in the kitchen.

With careful planning and mindful eating, you can maintain a balanced diet that promotes long-term wellness.

Veggie Omelet

Ingredients:

1. 2 large eggs
2. 1/4 cup diced bell peppers
3. 1/4 cup diced onions
4. 1/4 cup spinach leaves
5. 1 tablespoon olive oil
6. Black pepper and fresh herbs (optional, to taste)

Instructions:

1. In a bowl, whisk the eggs until well beaten.

2. Heat the olive oil in a non-stick skillet over medium heat.

3. Add the bell peppers and onions, cooking until they are tender, about 3-4 minutes.

4. Add the spinach leaves and cook until wilted, about 1-2 minutes.

5. Pour the beaten eggs over the vegetables in the skillet.

6. Cook until the eggs are set, about 2-3 minutes. Fold the omelet in half and slide it onto a plate.

7. Season with black pepper and fresh herbs if desired.

Nutritional Information (per serving):

1. Calories: 250
2. Protein: 14g
3. Carbohydrates: 5g
4. Fiber: 2g
5. Sugars: 2g
6. Fat: 20g
7. Sodium: 140mg

Serving Size: 1 omelet

Cooking Time: 10 minutes

Oatmeal with Fresh Berries

Ingredients:

1.   1/2 cup rolled oats
2.   1 cup water or unsweetened almond milk
3.   1/2 cup mixed berries (strawberries, blueberries, raspberries)
4.   1 tablespoon honey or maple syrup (optional)
5.   1/4 teaspoon ground cinnamon

Instructions:

1. In a small saucepan, bring the water or almond milk to a boil.

2. Stir in the rolled oats and reduce the heat to a simmer.

3. Cook for about 5 minutes, stirring occasionally, until the oats are soft and have absorbed most of the liquid.

4. Pour the cooked oatmeal into a bowl and top with fresh berries.

5. Drizzle with honey or maple syrup if desired, and sprinkle with ground cinnamon.

Nutritional Information (per serving):

1. Calories: 200

2. Protein: 5g

3. Carbohydrates: 40g

4. Fiber: 6g

5. Sugars: 15g

6. Fat: 3g

7. Sodium: 0mg

Serving Size: 1 bowl

Cooking Time: 10 minutes

Greek Yogurt Parfait

Ingredients:

1. 1 cup plain Greek yogurt (low sodium)
2. 1/2 cup granola (low sodium)
3. 1/2 cup mixed berries (blueberries, strawberries, raspberries)
4. 1 tablespoon honey

Instructions:

1. In a parfait glass or bowl, layer 1/3 cup of Greek yogurt.

2. Add a layer of granola followed by a layer of mixed berries.

3. Repeat the layers until all ingredients are used.

4. Drizzle the top with honey.

Nutritional Information (per serving):

1. Calories: 300
2. Protein: 15g
3. Carbohydrates: 50g
4. Fiber: 7g
5. Sugars: 25g
6. Fat: 7g
7. Sodium: 50mg

Serving Size: 1 parfait   **Cooking Time**: 5 minutes

Avocado Toast

Ingredients:

1. 1 slice whole grain bread (low sodium)
2. 1/2 ripe avocado
3. 1 teaspoon lemon juice
4. Black pepper and red pepper flakes (optional, to taste)

Instructions:

1. Toast the slice of whole grain bread to your desired crispiness.

2. In a small bowl, mash the avocado with a fork and mix in the lemon juice.

3. Spread the avocado mixture evenly over the toasted bread.

4. Sprinkle with black pepper and red pepper flakes if desired.

Nutritional Information (per serving):

1. Calories: 250
2. Protein: 5g
3. Carbohydrates: 30g
4. Fiber: 10g
5. Sugars: 1g
6. Fat: 15g
7. Sodium: 75mg

Serving Size: 1 slice   **Cooking Time:** 5 minutes

Smoothie Bowl

Ingredients:

1. 1 banana
2. 1/2 cup frozen mixed berries
3. 1/2 cup unsweetened almond milk
4. 1/4 cup plain Greek yogurt (low sodium)
5. 1 tablespoon chia seeds
6. 1/4 cup granola (low sodium)
7. Fresh fruit and nuts for topping (optional)

Instructions:

1. In a blender, combine the banana, frozen berries, almond milk, and Greek yogurt.

2. Blend until smooth and creamy.

3. Pour the smoothie into a bowl.

4. Top with chia seeds, granola, and any additional fresh fruit or nuts.

Nutritional Information (per serving):

1. Calories: 300

2. Protein: 10g

3. Carbohydrates: 60g

4. Fiber: 10g

5. Sugars: 30g

6. Fat: 7g

7. Sodium: 50mg

Serving Size: 1 bowl

Cooking Time: 5 minutes

Lunch Recipes in Relation to LOW SODIUM FOOD LIST 2024

Grilled Chicken Salad

Ingredients:

1. 1 boneless, skinless chicken breast (4 oz)
2. 4 cups mixed greens (spinach, arugula, and lettuce)
3. 1/2 cup cherry tomatoes, halved
4. 1/4 cup cucumber, sliced
5. 1/4 red onion, thinly sliced
6. 1/4 avocado, sliced
7. 2 tbsp olive oil
8. 1 tbsp balsamic vinegar
9. 1 tsp dried oregano
10. Black pepper to taste

Instructions:

1. Preheat the grill to medium-high heat.

2. Brush the chicken breast with 1 tbsp olive oil and sprinkle with dried oregano and black pepper.

3. Grill the chicken for 6-7 minutes on each side, or until fully cooked.

4. In a large bowl, combine mixed greens, cherry tomatoes, cucumber, red onion, and avocado.

5. Slice the grilled chicken and place on top of the salad.

6. Drizzle with remaining olive oil and balsamic vinegar. Toss gently to combine.

Nutritional Information (per serving):

1. Calories: 350
2. Protein: 30g
3. Carbohydrates: 12g
4. Fiber: 6g
5. Sugars: 5g
6. Fat: 20g
7. Sodium: 120mg

Serving Size: 1 salad

Cooking Time: 20 minutes

Quinoa Bowl with Roasted Vegetables

Ingredients:

1. 1 cup quinoa, rinsed
2. 2 cups water
3. 1 cup broccoli florets
4. 1 red bell pepper, sliced
5. 1 zucchini, sliced
6. 1 tbsp olive oil
7. 1 tsp garlic powder
8. 1/2 tsp smoked paprika
9. Black pepper to taste
10. 1/4 cup crumbled feta cheese (optional)
11. 1 tbsp fresh parsley, chopped

Instructions:

1. Preheat the oven to 400°F.

2. In a medium pot, bring water to a boil. Add quinoa, reduce heat to low, cover, and simmer for 15 minutes or until water is absorbed.

3. On a baking sheet, toss broccoli, bell pepper, and zucchini with olive oil, garlic powder, smoked paprika, and black pepper.

4. Roast vegetables in the oven for 20 minutes, or until tender and slightly charred.

5. In a large bowl, combine cooked quinoa and roasted vegetables. Top with feta cheese and fresh parsley.

Nutritional Information (per serving):

1. Calories: 350
2. Protein: 10g
3. Carbohydrates: 50g
4. Fiber: 8g
5. Sugars: 7g
6. Fat: 12g
7. Sodium: 150mg

Serving Size: 1 bowl

Cooking Time: 35 minutes

Turkey and Avocado Wrap

Ingredients:

1. 1 whole wheat tortilla
2. 4 slices low sodium turkey breast
3. 1/2 avocado, mashed
4. 1/4 cup shredded carrots
5. 1/4 cup spinach leaves
6. 1 tbsp Greek yogurt (plain, low sodium)
7. 1 tsp lemon juice
8. Black pepper to taste

Instructions:

1. In a small bowl, mix mashed avocado with lemon juice and black pepper.
2. Spread the avocado mixture over the tortilla.
3. Layer turkey slices, shredded carrots, and spinach leaves on top.
4. Drizzle with Greek yogurt.
5. Roll up the tortilla tightly, slice in half, and serve.

Nutritional Information (per serving):

1. Calories: 350

2. Protein: 20g

3. Carbohydrates: 30g

4. Fiber: 8g

5. Sugars: 3g

6. Fat: 15g

7. Sodium: 200mg

Serving Size: 1 wrap

Cooking Time: 10 minutes

Lentil and Vegetable Soup

Ingredients:

1. 1 cup dried green lentils, rinsed
2. 6 cups low sodium vegetable broth
3. 1 medium onion, chopped
4. 2 carrots, chopped
5. 2 celery stalks, chopped
6. 2 garlic cloves, minced
7. 1 tsp dried thyme
8. 1 tsp dried oregano
9. Black pepper to taste
10. 1 cup spinach leaves

Instructions:

1. In a large pot, heat a small amount of olive oil over medium heat. Add onion, carrots, and celery, and sauté until vegetables are softened, about 5 minutes.

2. Add garlic, thyme, and oregano, and cook for another minute.

3. Stir in lentils and vegetable broth. Bring to a boil.

4. Reduce heat to low, cover, and simmer for 30-35 minutes, or until lentils are tender.

5. Stir in spinach leaves and cook for an additional 5 minutes.

6. Season with black pepper to taste before serving.

Nutritional Information (per serving):

1. Calories: 250

2. Protein: 15g

3. Carbohydrates: 40g

4. Fiber: 15g

5. Sugars: 6g

6. Fat: 3g

7. Sodium: 100mg

Serving Size: 1 bowl (about 2 cups)

Cooking Time: 45 minutes

These lunch recipes are designed to be both nutritious and low in sodium, helping you maintain a healthy diet without compromising on flavor. By using fresh ingredients and avoiding processed foods, you can enjoy delicious meals that support your health goals.

Dinner Recipes (Low Sodium Food List 2024)

Baked Lemon Herb Salmon

Ingredients:

1. 4 salmon fillets (6 oz each)
2. 2 tablespoons olive oil
3. 2 tablespoons fresh lemon juice
4. 1 tablespoon fresh parsley, chopped
5. 1 tablespoon fresh dill, chopped
6. 2 cloves garlic, minced
7. 1/4 teaspoon black pepper
8. 1 lemon, thinly sliced

Instructions:

1. Preheat the oven to 375°F (190°C).

2. In a small bowl, mix olive oil, lemon juice, parsley, dill, garlic, and black pepper.

3. Place salmon fillets on a baking sheet lined with parchment paper.

4. Brush the olive oil mixture evenly over the salmon fillets.

5. Place lemon slices on top of each fillet.

6. Bake for 20-25 minutes or until the salmon is cooked through and flakes easily with a fork.

Nutritional Information (per serving):

1. Calories: 350
2. Protein: 30g
3. Carbohydrates: 2g
4. Fiber: 0g
5. Sugars: 0g
6. Fat: 23g
7. Sodium: 60mg

Serving Size: 1 fillet

Cooking Time: 25 minutes

Quinoa Stuffed Bell Peppers

Ingredients:

1. 4 large bell peppers (any color)
2. 1 cup quinoa, rinsed
3. 2 cups low sodium vegetable broth
4. 1 cup black beans, drained and rinsed
5. 1 cup corn kernels (fresh or frozen)
6. 1 cup diced tomatoes (no salt added)
7. 1 teaspoon cumin
8. 1 teaspoon paprika
9. 1/4 teaspoon black pepper
10. 1/4 cup fresh cilantro, chopped

Instructions:

1. Preheat the oven to 375°F (190°C).

2. Cut the tops off the bell peppers and remove the seeds and membranes.

3. In a medium saucepan, bring vegetable broth to a boil. Add quinoa, reduce heat, cover, and simmer for 15 minutes or until quinoa is cooked and broth is absorbed.

4. In a large bowl, combine cooked quinoa, black beans, corn, diced tomatoes, cumin, paprika, and black pepper.

5. Stuff each bell pepper with the quinoa mixture and place in a baking dish.

6. Cover with foil and bake for 25-30 minutes. Remove foil and bake for an additional 5 minutes.

7. Sprinkle with fresh cilantro before serving.

Nutritional Information (per serving):

1. Calories: 250
2. Protein: 10g
3. Carbohydrates: 45g
4. Fiber: 8g
5. Sugars: 8g
6. Fat: 4g
7. Sodium: 70mg

Serving Size: 1 stuffed bell pepper

Cooking Time: 35 minutes

Stir-Fried Tofu and Vegetables

Ingredients:

1. 14 oz firm tofu, drained and cubed
2. 2 tablespoons olive oil
3. 1 red bell pepper, sliced
4. 1 yellow bell pepper, sliced
5. 1 cup broccoli florets
6. 1 cup snow peas
7. 2 cloves garlic, minced
8. 1 tablespoon fresh ginger, minced
9. 2 tablespoons low sodium soy sauce
10. 1 tablespoon rice vinegar
11. 1/4 teaspoon red pepper flakes (optional)
12. 2 green onions, sliced

Instructions:

1. Heat 1 tablespoon of olive oil in a large skillet over medium-high heat. Add tofu cubes and cook until golden brown on all sides, about 5-7 minutes. Remove tofu from skillet and set aside.

2. Add the remaining olive oil to the skillet. Add bell peppers, broccoli, and snow peas. Stir-fry for 5-7 minutes until vegetables are tender-crisp.

3. Add garlic and ginger, and stir-fry for an additional 1 minute.

4. Return tofu to the skillet and add low sodium soy sauce, rice vinegar, and red pepper flakes if using. Stir to combine and cook for another 2-3 minutes.

5. Garnish with sliced green onions before serving.

Nutritional Information (per serving):

1. Calories: 220
2. Protein: 12g
3. Carbohydrates: 15g
4. Fiber: 4g
5. Sugars: 5g
6. Fat: 14g
7. Sodium: 180mg

Serving Size: 1 cup

Cooking Time: 20 minutes

Lentil and Vegetable Stew

Ingredients:

1. 1 cup green lentils, rinsed
2. 1 tablespoon olive oil
3. 1 large onion, diced
4. 2 carrots, diced
5. 2 celery stalks, diced
6. 3 cloves garlic, minced
7. 1 zucchini, diced
8. 1 can diced tomatoes (no salt added)
9. 4 cups low sodium vegetable broth
10. 1 teaspoon thyme
11. 1 teaspoon oregano
12. 1/4 teaspoon black pepper
13. 2 cups spinach, chopped

Instructions:

1. In a large pot, heat olive oil over medium heat. Add onion, carrots, and celery. Sauté for 5-7 minutes until vegetables are softened.

2. Add garlic and zucchini, and cook for another 2 minutes.

3. Stir in lentils, diced tomatoes, vegetable broth, thyme, oregano, and black pepper.

4. Bring to a boil, then reduce heat and simmer for 25-30 minutes until lentils are tender.

5. Stir in spinach and cook for an additional 5 minutes until wilted.

Nutritional Information (per serving):

1. Calories: 200
2. Protein: 12g
3. Carbohydrates: 35g
4. Fiber: 12g
5. Sugars: 8g
6. Fat: 4g
7. Sodium: 140mg

Serving Size: 1 cup

Cooking Time: 40 minutes

Apple Slices with Almond Butter

Ingredients:

1. 1 large apple
2. 2 tablespoons unsalted almond butter

Instructions:

1. Wash and core the apple, then slice it into thin wedges.

2. Spread the almond butter evenly on each apple slice.

Nutritional Information (per serving):

1. Calories: 200
2. Protein: 4g
3. Carbohydrates: 30g
4. Fiber: 5g
5. Sugars: 20g
6. Fat: 8g
7. Sodium: 0mg

Serving Size: 1 large apple with 2 tablespoons almond butter

Cooking Time: 5 minutes

Carrot and Cucumber Sticks with Hummus

Ingredients:

1. 1 large carrot
2. 1 cucumber
3. 1/4 cup low sodium hummus

Instructions:

1. Peel and slice the carrot and cucumber into sticks.
2. Serve the vegetable sticks with hummus on the side.

Nutritional Information (per serving):

1. Calories: 100
2. Protein: 2g
3. Carbohydrates: 15g
4. Fiber: 4g
5. Sugars: 6g
6. Fat: 4g
7. Sodium: 50mg

Serving Size: 1 large carrot, 1 cucumber, 1/4 cup hummus
Cooking Time: 10 minutes

Greek Yogurt with Berries

Ingredients:

1. 1 cup plain Greek yogurt (low sodium)
2. 1/2 cup mixed berries

Instructions:

1. Combine the Greek yogurt and mixed berries in a bowl.

2. Stir gently to mix.

Nutritional Information (per serving):

1. Calories: 150
2. Protein: 10g
3. Carbohydrates: 20g
4. Fiber: 3g
5. Sugars: 15g
6. Fat: 3g
7. Sodium: 60mg

Serving Size: 1 cup yogurt with 1/2 cup berries
Cooking Time: 5 minutes

Rice Cakes with Avocado

Ingredients:

1. 2 plain rice cakes
2. 1/2 avocado
3. A pinch of black pepper

Instructions:

1. Mash the avocado and spread it evenly on each rice cake.

2. Sprinkle with black pepper.

Nutritional Information (per serving):

1. Calories: 180
2. Protein: 3g
3. Carbohydrates: 25g
4. Fiber: 5g
5. Sugars: 0g
6. Fat: 10g
7. Sodium: 10mg

Serving Size: 2 rice cakes with 1/2 avocado

Cooking Time: 5 minutes

Air-Popped Popcorn

Ingredients:

1. 3 cups air-popped popcorn
2. 1 tablespoon olive oil
3. 1 teaspoon nutritional yeast

Instructions:

1. Toss the air-popped popcorn with olive oil.

2. Sprinkle with nutritional yeast.

Nutritional Information (per serving):

1. Calories: 120
2. Protein: 3g
3. Carbohydrates: 18g
4. Fiber: 4g
5. Sugars: 0g
6. Fat: 5g
7. Sodium: 0mg

Serving Size: 3 cups

Cooking Time: 5 minutes

Edamame

Ingredients:

1. 1 cup shelled edamame
2. 1 teaspoon olive oil
3. A pinch of sea salt

Instructions:

1. Steam the edamame until tender.

2. Drizzle with olive oil and sprinkle with sea salt.

Nutritional Information (per serving):

1. Calories: 130
2. Protein: 11g
3. Carbohydrates: 9g
4. Fiber: 4g
5. Sugars: 2g
6. Fat: 5g
7. Sodium: 50mg

Serving Size: 1 cup

Cooking Time: 10 minutes

Celery Sticks with Cream Cheese

Ingredients:

1. 2 celery stalks

2. 2 tablespoons low-fat cream cheese

Instructions:

1. Cut the celery into sticks.

2. Fill each celery stick with cream cheese.

Nutritional Information (per serving):

1. Calories: 100

2. Protein: 3g

3. Carbohydrates: 5g

4. Fiber: 2g

5. Sugars: 3g

6. Fat: 7g

7. Sodium: 75mg

Serving Size: 2 celery stalks with 2 tablespoons cream cheese

Cooking Time: 5 minutes

Cottage Cheese with Pineapple

Ingredients:

1. 1/2 cup low sodium cottage cheese
2. 1/2 cup pineapple chunks

Instructions:

1. Mix the cottage cheese and pineapple chunks in a bowl.

Nutritional Information (per serving):

1. Calories: 140
2. Protein: 12g
3. Carbohydrates: 15g
4. Fiber: 1g
5. Sugars: 13g
6. Fat: 3g
7. Sodium: 150mg

Serving Size: 1/2 cup cottage cheese with 1/2 cup pineapple

Cooking Time: 5 minutes

Cherry Tomatoes with Mozzarella

Ingredients:

1. 1 cup cherry tomatoes
2. 1/2 cup low sodium mozzarella balls

Instructions:

1. Combine cherry tomatoes and mozzarella balls in a bowl.

Nutritional Information (per serving):

1. Calories: 150
2. Protein: 10g
3. Carbohydrates: 7g
4. Fiber: 2g
5. Sugars: 5g
6. Fat: 10g
7. Sodium: 100mg

Serving Size: 1 cup tomatoes with 1/2 cup mozzarella

Cooking Time: 5 minutes

Almonds and Raisins Mix

Ingredients:

1. 1/4 cup unsalted almonds
2. 1/4 cup raisins

Instructions:

1. Mix almonds and raisins together in a bowl.

Nutritional Information (per serving):

1. Calories: 200
2. Protein: 6g
3. Carbohydrates: 28g
4. Fiber: 4g
5. Sugars: 18g
6. Fat: 10g
7. Sodium: 0mg

Serving Size: 1/2 cup mix

Cooking Time: 2 minutes

Baked Sweet Potato Chips

Ingredients:

1. 1 large sweet potato
2. 1 tablespoon olive oil
3. A pinch of paprika

Instructions:

1. Preheat the oven to 400°F.

2. Slice the sweet potato thinly and toss with olive oil and paprika.

3. Spread on a baking sheet and bake for 20 minutes.

Nutritional Information (per serving):

1. Calories: 160
2. Protein: 2g
3. Carbohydrates: 28g
4. Fiber: 4g
5. Sugars: 8g
6. Fat: 6g
7. Sodium: 30mg

Serving Size: 1 large sweet potato

Cooking Time: 25 minutes

Oatmeal with Banana and Cinnamon

Ingredients:

1. 1/2 cup rolled oats
2. 1 cup water
3. 1/2 banana
4. 1/4 teaspoon cinnamon

Instructions:

1. Cook the oats with water according to package instructions.

2. Slice the banana and top the oatmeal with banana slices and cinnamon.

Nutritional Information (per serving):

1. Calories: 200
2. Protein: 5g
3. Carbohydrates: 40g
4. Fiber: 5g
5. Sugars: 12g
6. Fat: 3g
7. Sodium: 0mg

Serving Size: 1 bowl

Cooking Time: 10 minutes

Sliced Bell Peppers with Guacamole

Ingredients:

1. 1 bell pepper
2. 1/4 cup guacamole

Instructions:

1. Slice the bell pepper into strips.
2. Serve with guacamole on the side.

Nutritional Information (per serving):

1. Calories: 150
2. Protein: 2g
3. Carbohydrates: 10g
4. Fiber: 5g
5. Sugars: 4g
6. Fat: 10g
7. Sodium: 100mg

Serving Size: 1 bell pepper with 1/4 cup guacamole

Cooking Time: 5 minutes

Yogurt with Honey and Walnuts

Ingredients:

1. 1 cup plain Greek yogurt
2. 1 tablespoon honey
3. 2 tablespoons unsalted walnuts

Instructions:

1. Mix the yogurt with honey.
2. Top with walnuts.

Nutritional Information (per serving):

1. Calories: 200
2. Protein: 10g
3. Carbohydrates: 20g
4. Fiber: 2g
5. Sugars: 18g
6. Fat: 8g
7. Sodium: 50mg

Serving Size: 1 cup yogurt with toppings
Cooking Time: 5 minutes

Turkey and Avocado Roll-Ups

Ingredients:

1. 4 slices low sodium turkey breast
2. 1/2 avocado
3. 1 teaspoon lemon juice

Instructions:

1. Mash the avocado with lemon juice.

2. Spread the mixture on turkey slices and roll up.

Nutritional Information (per serving):

1. Calories: 150
2. Protein: 15g

Chapter 9: Dining Out Tips

Choosing Low Sodium Options at Restaurants

Eating out while adhering to a low sodium diet can be challenging, but with careful planning and informed choices, you can enjoy restaurant meals without compromising your health goals. Begin by researching restaurants that offer low sodium options or are willing to accommodate special dietary requests.

Many establishments now provide nutritional information on their websites, making it easier to evaluate menu items before you arrive. Choose places known for their fresh, made-to-order dishes rather than those relying heavily on processed or pre-packaged ingredients.

When you arrive at the restaurant, don't hesitate to ask your server for recommendations or modifications to menu items. Most restaurants are accustomed to catering to various dietary needs and will gladly help you find suitable options.

Request dishes to be prepared without added salt and inquire about cooking methods. Opt for grilled, baked, or steamed items rather than fried or breaded foods, as these typically contain less sodium.

Salads can be a great low sodium choice if you are mindful of the ingredients and dressings. Ask for dressings on the side so you can control the amount used, or request a simple olive oil and vinegar mix. Avoid high sodium toppings such as croutons, bacon bits, and processed cheese.

Instead, load up on fresh vegetables and lean proteins like grilled chicken or shrimp. Customizing your salad ensures you enjoy a nutritious meal without unnecessary sodium.

Soups are often high in sodium, so it's best to avoid them unless the restaurant offers a specific low sodium option. Similarly, be cautious with sauces and gravies, which can add significant amounts of sodium to your meal.

Request these to be served on the side, allowing you to add only a small amount or skip them altogether. Lemon, fresh herbs, and spices can enhance the flavor of your meal without adding extra sodium.

For main courses, choose simple dishes that highlight fresh ingredients. Grilled fish, chicken, or lean meats paired with steamed vegetables or a side salad are usually safe bets.

Avoid entrees with heavy sauces, marinades, or breading, as these can be hidden sources of sodium. If the restaurant offers a build-your-own option, take advantage of it to customize a meal that fits your dietary needs.

When it comes to side dishes, steer clear of those that are typically high in sodium, such as fries, mashed potatoes, and rice pilaf. Instead, opt for steamed vegetables, a baked potato (request it without salt), or a side salad.

Many restaurants will accommodate a request for no added salt if you inform them of your dietary requirements in advance. This proactive approach can help ensure your meal is prepared according to your specifications.

Desserts at restaurants can be tricky, as many contain hidden sodium. Fresh fruit, sorbet, or a small serving of a simple dessert like plain cheesecake may be lower in sodium than options like cakes, pies, or pastries.

Again, don't hesitate to ask your server for details about the ingredients and preparation methods. By making thoughtful choices and communicating your needs clearly, you can enjoy dining out while maintaining your low sodium lifestyle.

Customizing Orders to Reduce Sodium

When dining out, reducing sodium intake requires thoughtful customization of your orders. Begin by researching the restaurant's menu in advance if possible, identifying dishes that are likely to be lower in sodium.

Option for fresh, whole foods such as salads, grilled meats, and steamed vegetables rather than dishes that are fried or heavily sauced. Choosing simpler preparations allows for greater control over sodium content.

When you arrive at the restaurant, don't hesitate to ask the server detailed questions about the dishes. Inquire about how the food is prepared and if it is possible to request no added salt. Most restaurants are accommodating and will make adjustments to meet dietary needs.

Request sauces and dressings on the side, so you can control the amount used. This simple step can significantly reduce the sodium content of your meal.

Another effective strategy is to substitute side dishes that are typically high in sodium with healthier options.

For example, replace French fries or mashed potatoes with a side salad or steamed vegetables. When ordering salads, ask for oil and vinegar on the side instead of premade dressings, which are often high in sodium. If the restaurant offers a baked potato, request it plain and add your own toppings sparingly.

Portion control also plays a crucial role in managing sodium intake. Restaurant portions are often larger than necessary, which can contribute to consuming more sodium. Consider sharing an entrée with a dining companion or immediately packing half of your meal to take home.

This not only helps reduce sodium intake but also prevents overeating. Additionally, starting with a small appetizer or soup can help moderate your overall consumption.

Be mindful of hidden sources of sodium in menu items. Dishes that contain processed ingredients, such as deli meats, cheeses, and bread, are likely to be high in sodium. Choose dishes that highlight fresh, whole ingredients instead.

For example, opt for a grilled chicken breast over a chicken sandwich, and avoid dishes that are heavily seasoned or brined.

If possible, request that the kitchen use fresh herbs and spices instead of salt to enhance the flavor of your meal.

Drinks can also be a source of hidden sodium. Avoid sodas and other flavored beverages that may contain added sodium. Stick to water, herbal teas, or unsweetened beverages.

If you enjoy alcoholic drinks, opt for wine or beer over mixed drinks, as these can also contain high levels of sodium depending on the mixers used. Always ask about the ingredients in cocktails and avoid those with pre-made mixes.

Finally, stay informed and be proactive in communicating your dietary needs. If you dine out frequently, consider visiting restaurants that are known for accommodating special dietary requirements.

Building a relationship with the staff at your favorite restaurants can make it easier to customize your orders and ensure they understand your low sodium needs. By taking these steps, you can enjoy dining out without compromising your commitment to a low sodium diet.

Understanding Restaurant Menus

When dining out, understanding restaurant menus is crucial for maintaining a low sodium diet. Restaurants often use salt liberally to enhance flavor, preserve food, and entice customers.

By becoming familiar with common menu items and preparation methods, you can make informed choices that align with your dietary goals. Look for menu descriptions that mention words like "grilled," "steamed," "baked," or "roasted," as these cooking methods typically use less salt compared to fried or sautéed dishes.

One of the most effective strategies is to ask for modifications to your meal. Don't hesitate to request that your food be prepared without added salt. Most restaurants are willing to accommodate dietary restrictions if you communicate your needs clearly.

Request sauces and dressings on the side, as these can be major sources of hidden sodium. This allows you to control the amount you use or avoid them altogether.

Opting for fresh, whole foods is another way to minimize sodium intake while dining out. Choose dishes that feature fresh vegetables, lean proteins, and whole grains.

Salads, grilled fish, or a simple chicken breast with steamed vegetables are generally safer options. Avoid dishes with processed ingredients such as cured meats, cheeses, and breaded items, which are often high in sodium.

Pay close attention to the appetizers and sides offered on the menu. These can often contain just as much sodium as the main courses. Items like soups, bread, and dips are usually loaded with salt.

Instead, consider starting your meal with a fresh salad, but be cautious of the dressing. Ask for olive oil and vinegar on the side, or opt for a lemon wedge to add flavor without the sodium.

Beverages can also be a hidden source of sodium. Stick to water, unsweetened tea, or coffee. Avoid soft drinks, flavored waters, and alcoholic beverages that can contribute to your sodium intake. If you enjoy a cocktail, ask for it to be made with fresh ingredients and skip the salted rim.

When choosing a restaurant, consider looking up the menu online beforehand. Many restaurants now provide nutritional information on their websites, which can help you plan your meal in advance.

If nutritional information isn't available, look for menu items that are described with fresh, wholesome ingredients and avoid those with heavy sauces or dressings.

Lastly, it's important to remain mindful of portion sizes. Restaurants are known for serving large portions, which can inadvertently lead to higher sodium consumption. Consider sharing a meal with a friend or asking for a to-go box when your food arrives, so you can portion out a reasonable serving and save the rest for later.

By making thoughtful choices and asking the right questions, you can enjoy dining out while adhering to your low sodium diet and maintaining your health goals.

Chapter 10: Maintaining a Low Sodium Lifestyle

Strategies for LongTerm Success

Maintaining a low sodium lifestyle requires a dedicated approach, ensuring that dietary choices support long-term health goals. It's essential to be mindful of the foods we consume daily, opting for fresh produce, lean proteins, and whole grains.

This approach minimizes sodium intake while providing essential nutrients and flavors. Fresh fruits and vegetables, naturally low in sodium, are the foundation of a heart-healthy diet.

Incorporating a variety of colors and types ensures a diverse nutrient intake, supporting overall health and well-being. Leafy greens, berries, and root vegetables are excellent choices, offering vitamins, minerals, and antioxidants.

Protein is a crucial component of any diet, and choosing low-sodium options is vital for maintaining muscle mass and overall health. Fresh, unprocessed meats like chicken, turkey, and fish are preferable over processed alternatives.

These proteins provide essential amino acids without the added sodium found in deli meats, sausages, and canned fish. Plant-based proteins such as beans, lentils, and tofu are also excellent choices. They offer the benefits of fiber and other nutrients while keeping sodium levels in check.

Whole grains are another important element of a low-sodium lifestyle. Brown rice, quinoa, barley, and oats are excellent alternatives to refined grains. These whole grains retain their natural nutrients and fiber, promoting satiety and digestive health.

When choosing bread and cereals, it's crucial to read labels carefully, opting for products with minimal sodium content. Baking at home using low-sodium recipes can also help control sodium intake and allow for customization to suit personal tastes and nutritional needs.

Herbs and spices are essential tools for adding flavor to meals without relying on salt. Fresh herbs like basil, cilantro, and parsley, as well as dried spices like turmeric, cumin, and paprika, can transform dishes while keeping sodium levels low.

Experimenting with different combinations can create exciting and delicious meals, reducing the temptation to reach for the salt shaker.

Vinegars, lemon juice, and other acidic ingredients can also enhance flavors and make dishes more vibrant.

Awareness of hidden sodium sources is crucial for long-term success. Many packaged and processed foods contain high levels of sodium, even those that may not taste particularly salty. Sauces, dressings, soups, and snacks are common culprits.

Reading labels and choosing low-sodium or sodium-free options can significantly reduce daily intake. Cooking from scratch is another effective strategy, allowing for complete control over ingredients and sodium content. This practice not only reduces sodium intake but also encourages healthier eating habits overall.

Dining out can be challenging when maintaining a low-sodium lifestyle, but it's not impossible. Choosing restaurants that offer customizable menu options or explicitly low-sodium dishes can help.

Communicating dietary needs to the server and requesting modifications, such as no added salt or sauces on the side, can make a significant difference.

Being mindful of portion sizes and opting for fresh, whole foods when possible ensures that dining out remains an enjoyable experience without compromising health goals.

Lastly, staying informed and connected with supportive communities can make maintaining a low-sodium lifestyle more manageable.

Joining groups, whether online or in-person, provides access to shared experiences, recipes, and tips. Keeping abreast of new research and food product developments, such as the Low Sodium Food List 2024, can offer valuable insights and options.

Embracing a proactive and informed approach helps sustain long-term success, ensuring that a low-sodium lifestyle becomes a permanent and beneficial part of daily life.

Staying Motivated and Consistent

Maintaining a low-sodium lifestyle requires dedication, and staying motivated and consistent is crucial for success. The journey often begins with understanding the profound impact of sodium on health.

Sodium, while essential in small amounts, can lead to various health issues when consumed excessively, including hypertension, heart disease, and stroke.

Embracing a low-sodium diet can significantly improve health and well-being, making the effort worthwhile. The benefits of reduced sodium intake can be a powerful motivator, offering a clear goal to work towards.

To stay motivated, it is important to remember the reasons behind the dietary changes. Reflecting on personal health goals, such as reducing blood pressure or improving cardiovascular health, can reinforce the commitment to a low-sodium diet.

Setting specific, achievable goals can also help maintain focus and provide a sense of accomplishment as each milestone is reached.

Additionally, keeping a journal to track progress can serve as a tangible reminder of how far one has come and the benefits experienced along the way.

Consistency in a low-sodium lifestyle involves integrating new habits into daily routines. This can be challenging, especially when faced with the convenience of processed and fast foods, which are often high in sodium.

Preparing meals at home using fresh ingredients is a key strategy. Learning to read food labels meticulously is essential, as it helps identify hidden sources of sodium. Opting for fresh fruits, vegetables, lean proteins, and whole grains can naturally reduce sodium intake while providing essential nutrients.

Exploring new recipes and cooking methods can make the transition to a low-sodium diet more enjoyable. Experimenting with herbs, spices, and other sodium-free seasonings can enhance the flavor of dishes without the need for added salt.

Finding low-sodium versions of favorite foods or creating homemade alternatives can also help satisfy cravings without compromising the dietary goals.

Sharing meals with family and friends who support the low-sodium lifestyle can create a positive, encouraging environment.

Social support plays a significant role in maintaining motivation and consistency. Joining a community of individuals who share similar dietary goals can provide encouragement, share tips and recipes, and offer accountability.

Online forums, local support groups, or even social media platforms can connect individuals with a network of support. Having a support system can make the journey less isolating and more manageable, as members can inspire each other to stay on track.

Overcoming challenges and setbacks is a part of any lifestyle change. It is important to approach these moments with a positive mindset and resilience. Understanding that occasional slip-ups are normal and not a reason to abandon the low-sodium lifestyle can prevent feelings of discouragement.

Instead, viewing setbacks as opportunities to learn and grow can strengthen commitment. Developing strategies to handle difficult situations, such as dining out or attending social events, can also help maintain consistency.

Ultimately, the key to staying motivated and consistent with a low-sodium lifestyle lies in making sustainable changes and finding joy in the process. Celebrating small victories and appreciating the health benefits can reinforce positive behavior.

With time, the new habits will become second nature, making it easier to maintain the low-sodium lifestyle. The journey may have its challenges, but the long-term rewards of better health and well-being make it a worthwhile endeavor.

Monitoring Your Progress

Embarking on a low-sodium lifestyle requires dedication and awareness, but the rewards for your health are immeasurable. Monitoring your progress is essential to ensure that you're on the right path and making the necessary adjustments as you go along.

It starts with understanding your daily sodium intake and setting realistic goals. Keeping a detailed food diary can help you track what you eat and identify areas where you might be consuming more sodium than intended. This record-keeping allows you to see patterns in your diet and make informed choices to stay within your sodium limits.

One of the key aspects of maintaining a low-sodium lifestyle is becoming adept at reading food labels. Many processed foods contain hidden sodium, even those that don't taste salty. Learning to decode labels and recognize terms like "sodium," "salt," "soda," and "Na" can help you avoid high-sodium products.

Over time, this skill becomes second nature, and you'll be able to quickly identify healthier options at the grocery store.

Additionally, it's beneficial to familiarize yourself with the sodium content of common foods, so you can make smarter choices when eating out or preparing meals at home.

Consistency is crucial when monitoring your progress. Regularly checking your sodium intake helps you stay accountable and motivated. You might consider using apps or digital tools designed to track nutritional information, as they can provide real-time feedback and make the process more manageable.

These tools often come with databases of foods and their sodium content, making it easier to plan meals and snacks that fit into your low-sodium regimen. The convenience of having this information at your fingertips can be a significant factor in your success.

Support from friends, family, or a community of like-minded individuals can also play a vital role in maintaining your low-sodium lifestyle. Sharing your journey with others can provide encouragement and accountability.

Joining support groups, either online or in person, can offer a sense of camaraderie and the opportunity to exchange tips and recipes. When those around you understand and support your dietary choices, it becomes easier to stay on track and resist temptations.

It's important to celebrate your successes along the way, no matter how small they may seem. Recognizing your progress reinforces your commitment and boosts your morale.

Whether it's consistently staying within your sodium limits for a week, discovering a delicious low-sodium recipe, or feeling physically better, these milestones are worth acknowledging. Celebrating achievements helps maintain a positive mindset and keeps you focused on your long-term goals.

Adjustments are inevitable as you navigate a low-sodium lifestyle. You may find that certain foods or habits need to be altered as you gain more insight into your body's needs and responses. Flexibility and a willingness to adapt are essential.

Listening to your body and being open to change ensures that your low-sodium diet remains effective and sustainable. This might mean experimenting with different spices and herbs to add flavor without salt or finding new, low-sodium products that suit your taste and nutritional requirements.

Reflecting on your journey periodically helps reinforce the benefits of a low-sodium diet and reminds you why you started.

Take time to consider how far you've come, the challenges you've overcome, and the positive changes you've experienced. This reflection not only solidifies your commitment but also helps you appreciate the journey itself.

Monitoring your progress isn't just about keeping track of numbers; it's about understanding and appreciating the impact of your efforts on your overall health and well-being.

CONCLUSION

In the journey toward a healthier lifestyle, embracing a low-sodium diet stands out as a significant and impactful choice. As you navigate the realm of dietary changes, the importance of a low-sodium food list becomes increasingly clear.

It serves as a guiding compass, helping you make informed decisions that support your overall well- being.

The dedication to reducing sodium intake is not merely about following a list; it's about committing to a healthier way of living, where each choice contributes to long-term health benefits.

Adopting a low-sodium diet can initially seem daunting, but with the right resources and mindset, it becomes a manageable and rewarding endeavor.

The 2024 low-sodium food list is an essential tool in this process, offering a variety of options that align with your dietary goals.

By incorporating these foods into your daily routine, you take proactive steps toward reducing your sodium intake, thereby lowering the risk of hypertension, heart disease, and other related health issues.

This list empowers you to make better choices, fostering a sense of control over your health.

Over time, the benefits of a low-sodium diet become evident in numerous ways. Physically, you may notice improvements in blood pressure, reduced bloating, and an overall sense of well-being. These changes are a testament to the positive impact of consistently choosing low-sodium foods.

Additionally, your palate will begin to adjust, finding satisfaction in the natural flavors of food rather than the overpowering taste of salt. This shift not only enhances your enjoyment of meals but also contributes to a healthier, more balanced diet.

The journey of reducing sodium intake is also an educational one. You become more aware of the hidden sodium in many processed and restaurant foods, leading to more thoughtful eating habits.

This knowledge empowers you to advocate for healthier options, both for yourself and within your community. Sharing what you've learned with others can inspire them to embark on their own low-sodium journey, creating a ripple effect of healthier choices and improved well-being.

Maintaining a low-sodium diet is not without its challenges, but each obstacle overcome is a step toward a healthier future. Whether it's finding new recipes, adapting favorite dishes, or making conscious choices when dining out, every effort counts.

The commitment to a low-sodium lifestyle is a testament to your dedication to your health and quality of life. It reflects a willingness to prioritize long-term benefits over short-term conveniences, a decision that yields profound rewards over time.

As you reflect on your progress, it's important to recognize and celebrate your achievements. Each day that you adhere to a low-sodium diet is a victory for your health. The discipline and mindfulness required to make these choices contribute to a stronger, more resilient you.

By focusing on the positive changes and the benefits you experience, you reinforce your commitment to this lifestyle. The journey may have its ups and downs, but the overall trajectory is one of improved health and well-being.

In the end, the low-sodium food list is more than just a guide; it's a foundation for a healthier way of life. By consistently choosing foods that align with this list, you build a diet that supports your health goals and enhances your quality of life.

The journey toward a low-sodium lifestyle is a continuous one, marked by learning, growth, and positive change. With each choice you make, you contribute to a healthier, more vibrant future, embracing the benefits of a low-sodium diet and the empowerment it brings.

www.ingramcontent.com/pod-product-compliance
Lightning Source LLC
Chambersburg PA
CBHW051554250726
48653CB00004BA/1154